"Cedar's book humanizes the work with older adults beyond imagination. It not only inspired and encouraged me to do creative work with every living being, but I also found myself laughing and crying while reading it, as if I was watching a movie or a theatre piece. The book is written with enthusiasm and clarity: It describes the challenges and achievements of doing creative group work with people suffering from dementia, old age, and loneliness with utmost sincerity, enlightening depth, and a passionate desire to touch the reader's heart."

—**Professor Susana Pendzik, Ph.D., RDT,** *Tel Hai Academic College, Hebrew University of Jerusalem*

"In the field of dementia care we're always looking for additional ways to stimulate our groups. Once upon a time there was only music therapy and exercises. This book is fascinating, an easy read but also scientific, well versed in theoretical data and examples from life, while encouraging a new generation to get on the wagon and join in doing psychodrama. It not only adds a whole new field to our toolbox, but in line with the Melabev philosophy, accents what they can do, not what is lost; relates to them with dignity and uses the interaction within the group to build a safe, loving, support system."

—**Leah Abramowitz, M.S.W.**, *co-founder of Melabev, recipient of the Jerusalem Prize and the Builders of Zion Prize*

"This inspiring book authored by a true expert shows convincingly how a group of older adults suffering cognitive decline, Alzheimer's disease and other dementias responded individually and in group settings to a series of exercises clearly described in each part. It is amazing to find out how seniors with various cognitive impairments responded to a wide range of psychodrama techniques wonderfully explained in the book."

—**Soledad Ballesteros, Ph.D.**, *emeritus professor of Basic Psychology, Universidad Nacional de Educación a Distancia, Madrid*

Group Psychodrama for Dementia, Old Age, and Loneliness

Group Psychodrama for Dementia, Old Age, and Loneliness offers a fresh approach for professionals working with older individuals by employing new and exciting custom methodologies in psychodrama, particularly for clients with Alzheimer's disease or other forms of dementia.

This book offers a general explanation of the use of psychodrama by giving an overview of the therapeutic use of drama in all its forms, clearly explaining the concepts and methods, and describing the rationale of every intervention while also following a group over six years with precious documentation of the group process. It addresses the main concerns of those who suffer from dementia – adjusting to a new and changing level of functioning, fostering a sense of belonging, preserving their innate dignity, and redefining relationships and roles.

This practical guide will help therapists, social workers, family and other caregivers, teachers, and medical professionals working with older clients seeking comfort from the loneliness of old age and dementia using group psychodrama.

Tzippi Cedar, M.A.E., is a psychodramatist who deals with loss, loneliness, growth and self-efficacy. She teaches and works with therapists, social, geriatric and medical staff, teachers, parents, singles, children, adolescents and Holocaust survivors.

Group Psychodrama for Dementia, Old Age, and Loneliness

Trusting the Process

Tzippi Cedar

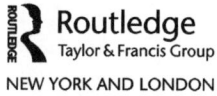
Routledge
Taylor & Francis Group

NEW YORK AND LONDON

Designed cover image: by Shalom Lincoln Rosenberg

First published 2023
by Routledge
605 Third Avenue, New York, NY 10158

and by Routledge
4 Park Square, Milton Park, Abingdon, Oxon, OX14 4RN

Routledge is an imprint of the Taylor & Francis Group, an informa business

ISBN: 978-1-032-34359-4 (hbk)
ISBN: 978-1-032-34358-7 (pbk)
ISBN: 978-1-003-32170-5 (ebk)

DOI: 10.4324/9781003321705

Typeset in NewBaskerville
by Apex CoVantage, LLC

I would like to dedicate this book to:
my husband, Howie

our children:
Joseph and Vered Kellner Cedar
Dahlia and Naftali Jacobs
Noa and Ezra Cedar Press
Yoav and Einav Cedar
Yonatan and Meirav Cedar
Daniel and Tali Cedar

our grandchildren:
Amalia, Levy, Yemima,
Hodaya, Moria, Matan, Meirav, Itamar, Yinnon,
Gabriel, Tamara, Louise,
Shay, Maayan, Hallel, Omer,
Alon, Roeh, Michael, Lev Aryeh,
Petal, Shaked, Yeala, Arbel

The artist Shalom Lincoln Rosenberg who painted the jacket
of this book. The entire staff at the Melabev English Speaking
Center in Jerusalem and especially, the participants in our
psychodrama sessions.

Thanks to you all for enabling and Trusting My Process

Contents

PART VIII

The greatest gift we can give people is to give them the chance to create. This is one gift that turns the recipient into a giver. It gives them dignity. It shows them we trust them, have faith in them, and believe they are capable of great things.

Rabbi Lord Jonathan Sacks, (2020)
Judaism's Life-Changing Ideas,
Jerusalem, Maggid Books

About the Author

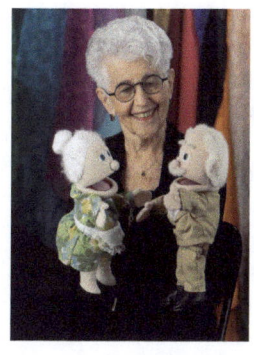 Tzippi Cedar is a psychodrama therapist who works with individuals and groups of all ages. Her rich career in drama education and therapy began over sixty years ago. She conducts psychodrama workshops, courses, supervision and therapy for parent groups, singles groups, post-trauma grief groups, cancer patients, medical staff, therapists, geriatric patients, second-generation Holocaust survivors, emotional first aid telephone volunteers, teachers, children, adolescents, social workers and geriatric workers. Her vast experience has taken her to hospitals, schools, teachers' colleges, universities and museums throughout Israel and the United States. She has brought drama as a learning and healing tool into classrooms from kindergarten through twelfth grade.

As a ventriloquist who performed with an educational puppet theatre in Israel and in the United States, she has reached children of all ages. She is still enchanting audiences, enabling deep communication and delivering important life-changing messages with her original custom-made *talking* puppets. Her innovative work with Alzheimer patients and senior citizens suffering from all forms of dementia and loneliness shows her ability to leap from theory to practice and bring energy, spontaneity and hope into the life of everyone she works with.

She was born in New York City in 1942 and moved to Jerusalem, Israel, in 1973. She is married to Professor Howard Cedar. They are the parents of six and the grandparents of twenty-four. This is her first book, and she is treating it like a great-grandchild.

About the Cover

The illustration on the cover was painted by Shalom Lincoln Rosenberg, a member of our psychodrama group who added color and dimension to our sessions. He passed away July 27, 2022 five days after I told him his painting would be the cover of this book and more of his artistic expression will be presented here.

He discovered his talent at the center and over these past few years has painted over 100 paintings that give him dignity and satisfaction. I chose this painting because it invites us to experience his inner world – his confusion as well as his desire to release feelings buried deep inside – so that he can feel more integrated with the world around him. These are some of the major goals of my group psychodrama work. He loved our sessions.

Following are a few examples of the artwork of Shalom Lincoln Rosenberg which are proudly displayed on the walls of our meeting room at the Melabev Center and in his home (Images 0.2–0.7).

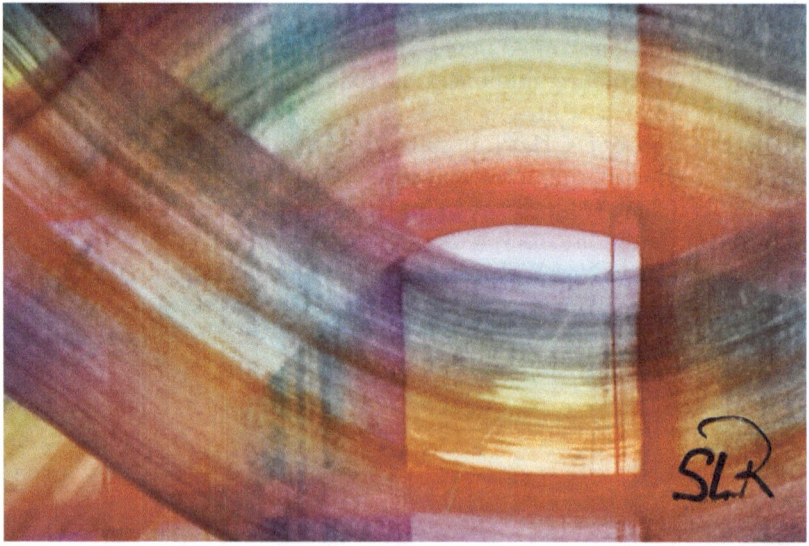

Image 0.2 Looking for Harmony

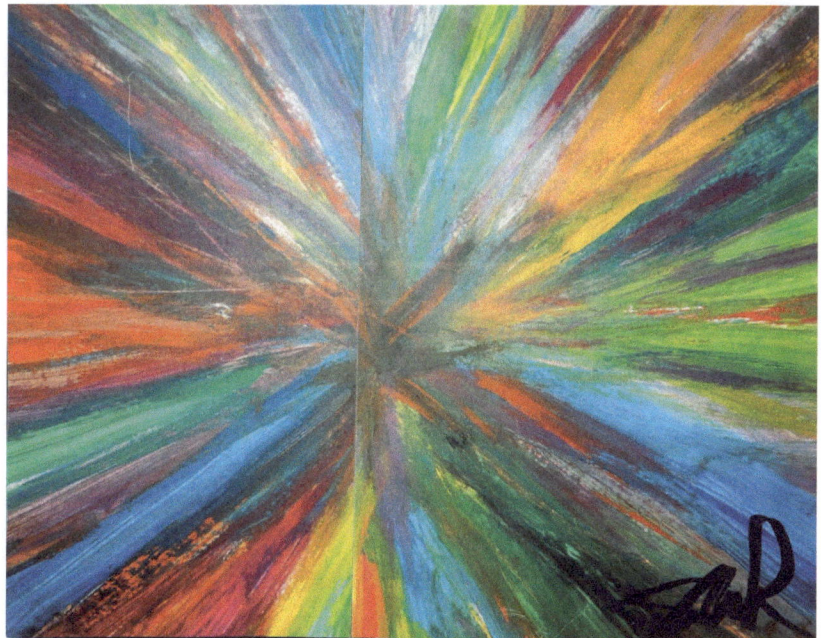

Image 0.3 Reaching for Joy

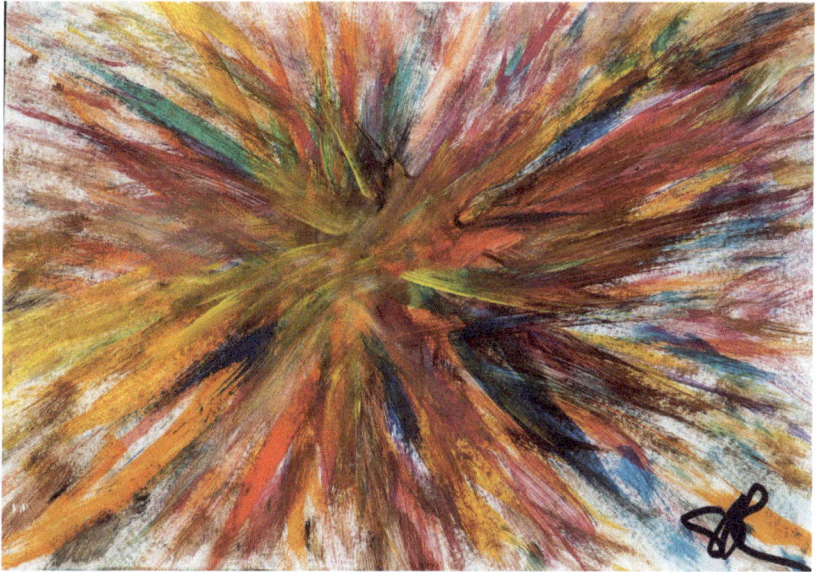

Image 0.4 My Meteor

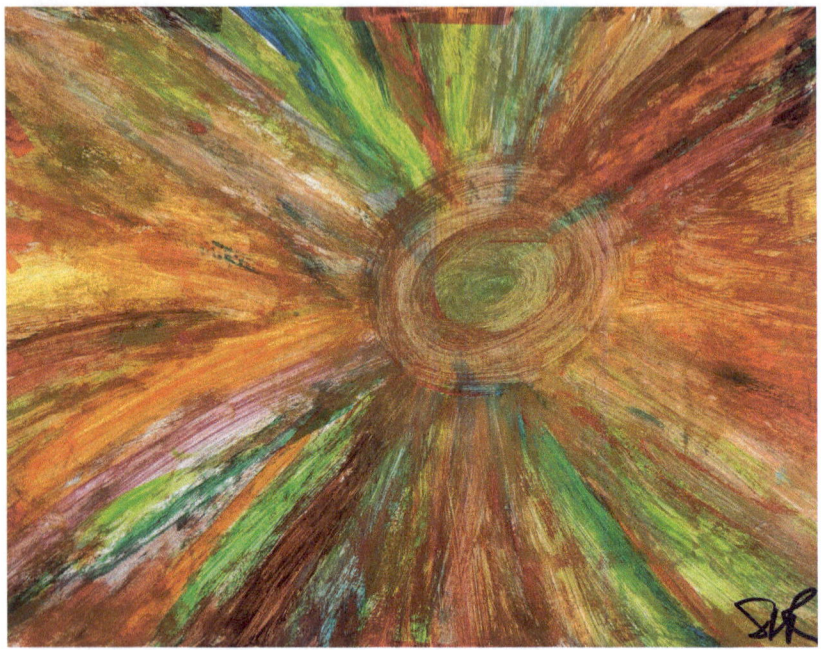

Image 0.5 Sun Rays on My Life

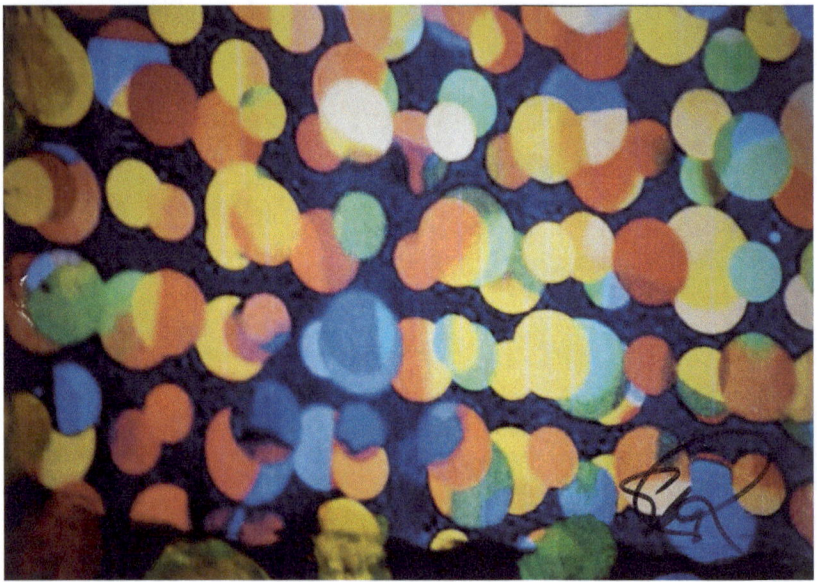

Image 0.6 Searching Through Movement

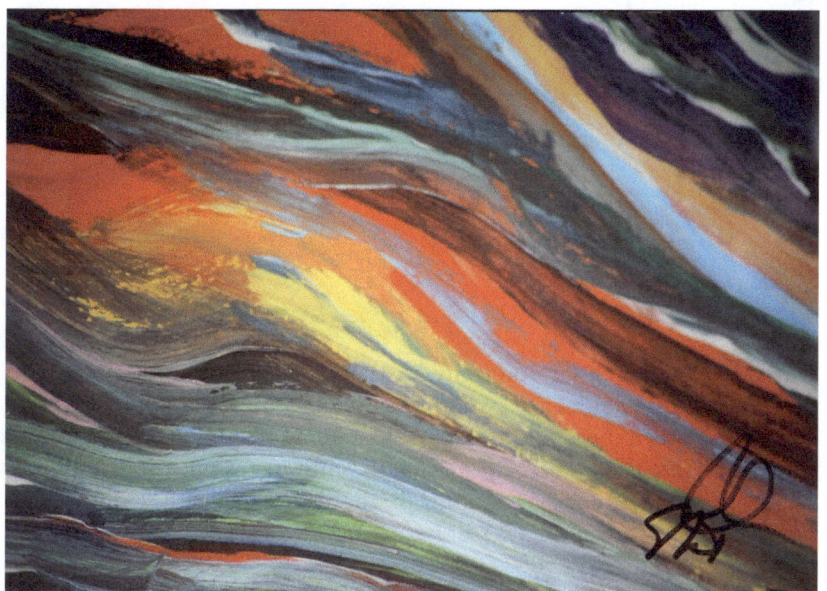

Image 0.7 Ups and Downs

Foreword

During the last decade, longevity has been increasing, and along with its benefits the health-care system of our society has to explore creative methodologies to better address the challenges of aging. However, along with longer life, we have also seen that the number of persons presenting symptoms of dementia is constantly on the rise. Faced with symptomatology whose standard model is still neurocognitive, we are inclined toward focusing primarily on the disabilities of the person rather than their remaining capacities and how we can enhance them.

Since significant research within the field of dementia has demonstrated that "emotional intelligence" still remains relatively active, it is clinically important to explore mechanisms to allow persons with dementia to use their emotional intelligence to enhance their self-efficacy. This concept has grown out of a social psychology construct of human agency. Self-efficacy plays a significant role in functionality (physical and cognitive).

In this book, you will read, learn and be able to apply a specific set of techniques based on the methodology of psychodrama that enhances the autonomy of persons with dementia. This book thus could allow health-care professionals, family members and caregivers to design creative strategies and conditions in the living environment of the person with dementia in order to rebuild and maintain a sense of self-efficacy, along with acknowledging the challenges arising from normal physiological and pathological changes in the trajectory of dementia. The methodologies discussed in this book would thus improve the quality of life of persons with dementia and their families. Enjoy! And learn.

Dr. Chariklia-|Tziraki Segal, MD., Ph.D.
Professor of Medical and Health Care Science

Preface

When I leave this world, I know that I am leaving behind six happily married children to incredible life partners, twenty-four beautiful, healthy, vital, amazing grandchildren and a husband who has been the greatest gift a woman could receive, over and over every day of our life together. They will all have wonderful memories of loving, living and laughing together. But what about the other "births"?!

What about the interactive exercises in the classroom that save children from anonymity and change their social lives, self-image and ability to communicate with themselves, others and their surroundings? What of the cohesive results of my interactive work on loneliness for people in all my groups? What about the action insights, through psychodrama, with all the clients and groups I have worked with over the years? What about the tools, the numerous workshops that I have given for all the educators, parents and people who deal with the development of children, by using drama in the classroom, camp, clubroom or home? What about all the work with the elderly, people with Alzheimer's disease and other forms of dementia? What about the work with Second-Generation Holocaust survivors? All the psychodrama groups I led? What about the work with cancer patients, with post-trauma grief groups? What about the singles' groups? What of the moments, those magical moments, when the truth is expressed effortlessly and authentically through using psychodramatic enactments in group settings? I would like all these moments to be remembered too.

I don't know who will read this book, but I know that all the people I have worked with for way over fifty years will understand the language and relive the spontaneous results of our experiential work, in the classrooms, clinics, auditoriums, living-rooms and improvised spaces. We worked together in groups, being creative, in order to bring about change in a dynamic, safe environment that facilitates growth, development and JOY!

So many have encouraged me to write it all down for others to learn how to use drama with children – of all ages. So, I am going to guide you in the language of *concretizing*, *enactment*, showing and yes, telling.

I am going to enable you to make people feel comfortable together, in a group, in a creative, spontaneous, healthy, vital, enabling environment. I will tell it through explanations, stories, a sharing of my experiences and description of exercises that you can use. My hope is that you too will be inspired to *trust the process*! I will be giving the theory behind the work and the rationale for choosing specific exercises with different populations. All of this work has been inspired by educators, psychologists, expressive art therapists, and mostly by the people I have worked with from ages 3 to 100! Through my interaction with all of these people, I have learned to trust the process.

This is all being written in the hope that you will read this book and want to work with people and you will flow with the process. That you will expand your language and use *empathy* and all the elements from the magic tool box of drama: the *mirroring, twinship, grandiosity, attunement* and deep *tele* – which I hope this book will help you discover and understand – and you will grow with the process.

This book was initially going to be a chapter in a book on how to be creative with children. The original title was *Drama with Mama* based on self-theory concepts taken from the relationship between a mother and child. These concepts were established by Heinz Kohut, an Austrian-born American psychoanalyst best known for his development of self-psychology. Four of his concepts that have really helped me in my work were among those just mentioned earlier: *empathy, mirroring, twinship and grandiosity*. The chapter grew into this detailed account of my work and my process with senior citizens at a Jerusalem day center called Melabev (see Appendix).

Acknowledgments

In Appreciation

Thank you to all my students over the years who have encouraged me to "write a book".

Thank you to the participants in this group who struggle so hard every minute of their days to be in their yes.

Thank you to the staff and volunteers at Melabev: Dvora, the dedicated director, whose inner wisdom affected and helped everyone at the center; Jackie the totally involved social worker; Michal, our empathic talented volunteer; Jennie, the incredible group leader who worked so professionally and devotedly to ensure our people were able to participate and benefit; and finally, Melabev's medical consultant, Chariklia, who became my mentor and whose knowledge and experience made her trust and inspire this process.

My thanks go to my astute readers Sherri Mandell and my sister Marion for their generosity with their time, thoroughness and talent.

This is my first book, and it has been my good fortune to find the best professionals to guide me and help me in this project.

My thanks to my photographer Elior, and his partner Dima at Damka Studio, for capturing this process with such sensitivity and confidence.

My thanks to Aloma, my incredible editor. She has become my friend and an integral part of trusting this process in every way.

I have discovered how fortunate I have been to work with Amanda and Katya at Routledge. You have both been my guides. At each stage you moved me forward with your genuine enthusiasm and prompt, professional, precise and warm instructions. You are both so beautiful inside and out and have made me feel so comfortable confident and . . . young.

My family gives me love, confidence and validation in everything I do! They know how thankful and proud I am to be their mother and grandmother.

My deepest thanks to my darling husband Howie who brought me to my YES at every stage of the process with this book and in our life through his wisdom, inspiring example and deep love.

So much to be thankful for!

Part I

Essential Background

Defining the Process

An Invitation to View a Session: The Forest

Let's start out with an illustration of a session that proves that one can do drama in all its forms to great effect with Alzheimer patients. This is like a trailer for a movie.

It is ten o'clock on a Tuesday morning. Eighteen senior citizens are sitting in a circle, waiting expectantly for their drama session with a gray-haired lady. She calls it psychodrama or drama therapy or just plain drama. She always begins with, "Today, we will do . . .". That's the key word – DO. What can eighteen people with dementia, diseases like Parkinson's and Alzheimer's, hearing and vision impairment and motor issues – DO? Let's take a peek at what transpires.

> We will use drama to do something really special. Today, we are not going to be people. We are not going to talk about our problems and issues. Today we are going to leave this room, this neighborhood, this city. We are going to arrive at a beautiful forest that we will create together. Were you ever in a forest?

I now launch into Guided Imagery.

> If you feel comfortable closing your eyes, it could help you visualize an amazing special forest that we are going to create in this room. If you don't, you certainly don't have to close your eyes. Do whatever is necessary to concentrate on creating a forest right here in this room. Right now, imagine a forest, very green. There are trees and plants of all sizes, all shades of green. We can hear the sounds of birds chirping, the movement of the water in the lake and the wind rustling in the trees. We can smell the fragrance of the different trees and shrubs. This is a peaceful, verdant place in nature. Now imagine, if you could be something in this forest, what would you choose to be?

DOI: 10.4324/9781003321705-1

We open our eyes. I say, "What are YOU in this forest?"

Here, as people from my Melabev group start speaking, one after another, I should emphasize that all the names of people in my groups have been changed to preserve their privacy.

Moe: (aged 98, and the most senior member of the group), says with immense distinction, "I am the oldest tree in the forest. I've seen everything. I am hardy and sturdy. No one is a stronger or older tree than I am. All these years and all my experiences have made me wise."

As the oldest member of our group his words carry great resonance.

Martin: "I'm a bench in the forest. People come to sit and rest on me and listen to the music of the concerts given here."

Herbie: (His Alzheimer's is advancing rapidly and he is terrified.) "I'm a turtle. My shell is protecting me."

Pauline: "I'm a rare mushroom. I will make everything you cook much more delicious."

Debra: (always complaining about the noise in the room, the chattering everything! Always telling everyone to shut up!) "I'm an owl. I observe everything that is going on. It is very quiet and serene, up here, on my branch high above the forest."

I have never seen her so calm.

Our forest is growing. Others begin to present their new roles as they identify with them.

"I am a tree house in big tree, for the children to play in."
"I am a bird."
"I am the stream flowing through the forest with cool refreshing water."

Now the more reticent join in: "I am a chipmunk . . . I am a bluebell . . . the wind . . . a worm . . . a sweet pretty bird . . . a deer . . . a frog . . . a fish, a pinecone, a gorilla, an eagle, a strong, unbreakable branch of a tree for children to swing on." We also meet a squirrel, the warm sun, even meat cooking on the barbeque, and so much more. We are creating an idyllic place.

I continue, "How do you feel in this forest we have created?"

Here are just a few of their statements that illustrate how they are transported into this fantasy.

"I feel safe."
"It's a beautiful day and it gives me great pleasure to see the children splashing in my water."

"I just want to be left alone, so I'll sit here and look at something beautiful – like these bluebells."

After everyone expresses what they are and how they feel in the forest, interactions are developed between them: the animals drink from the stream, the sun warms the animals and envelops the plants, the trees give shade and protection and provide a place for the children to swing and climb. The bigger animals take care of the vulnerable ones. It really is incredible. They do not want this session to end.

When asked, "What can we call this forest?" Debra, who is always grouchy and ornery says, to our utter amazement, "Let's call it, the *Family Forest*. We can take it all in and see the beauty in ourselves."

They interact so naturally and comfortably. This was a drama experience that gave people who are normally impatient, frustrated, unsure and ill-at-ease with themselves, calm, repose, aesthetics, and an uplifting experience.

This was a session that they remembered. It was transformative. When asked what they would like to take from this forest, their immediate response was: calmness, feeling relaxed, connected to nature, feeling beautiful, the flow of the water, the interaction with nature. I took their ability to transcend reality and benefit from this delicate fantasy. Despite their disabilities, their self-efficacy improved in this new process of engagement. This was obvious in the session. Somehow, I felt that they also went home feeling less lonely and more capable of involvement. I went home knowing that, Yes, you CAN do drama in all its forms with Alzheimer patients and lonely senior citizens.

So,. let's start from the beginning.

My Initiation

When I was asked to work at Melabev, a Jerusalem day center for the elderly who have Alzheimer's disease and other forms of dementia, I said, "NO! I have no experience with this population."

Then I thought, why not? I have lots of experience with group work and I love challenges. These people can be high functioning. You've seen how you can adapt psychodrama techniques to the classroom, work place, living room; you've seen how you can help people with disabilities, illness, post-trauma and many other populations. Surely you can adapt the method to this group. Not only that, but you're close to their age, so you know what their issues are. Almost everyone you know is dealing with someone in this population. Give it a try. As J.L. Moreno, the father of psychodrama, said, "Trust the Process."

So, I find myself working with a remarkable group at Melabev called the Challenge Group. Where will you find in one group people who were authors, heads of departments in hospitals and universities, a curator in a museum in New York, a designer of fabrics for haute couture fashion, a plumber, a rabbi, a rabbi's wife, teachers, a lonely housewife, a watchmaker, a handyman, an artist, a musician, survivors of the Holocaust and of Auschwitz, a psychiatrist, an electrical engineer – among others? I have so much to learn from them. On the spectrum, they are considered high functioning. They are not yet in the most advanced stages of Alzheimer's disease and they are, more or less, aware of their situation. This is difficult for them! As a result, our sessions were incredibly beneficial to their wellbeing, emotional stability, self-awareness and health. They were dealing with all the issues of aging, plus Alzheimer's, Parkinson's and Lewy bodies disease, varied degrees of dementia, as well as coping with the threat of what lay ahead for them. Above all, like many people whom I've met in my groups, they were dealing with loneliness. My best argument to myself was:

> You have witnessed so many people benefitting from group work in all of the drama methods, so maybe you can help this population too? Hopefully this group work will help create a quality of life that produces a sense of belonging and diminishes the loneliness that old age brings.

Hopefully, this group work will help create a quality of life that produces a sense of belonging and diminishes the loneliness that old age brings.

I am going to share my experience of doing psychodrama with this population. I will tell you what I learned from them and how it is possible to translate tools and techniques from psychodrama to their language and to their abilities and how they guided me in adapting the method to their special needs. I will include many of their responses, bring quotes from our sessions and, here and there, details of sessions will be elaborated so that you can see how interesting and exciting it is to work with people coping with dementia and other issues related to aging.

The documentation, of the sessions, is so valuable. I hope this will encourage you to work with this challenging and rewarding population. This book should also benefit family members, especially those who have become caregivers, who wish for a more sensitive, empathic, dignified interaction in their aging parents' lives. I will also share my frustrations, doubts and disappointments because that is something that anyone who works with this population will surely experience. Of course, this applies to anyone working with a group coping with loneliness and the need to feel comfortable and socially vital. Because their lives are filled with "no" we must affirm their "yes". But before doing that, we have to look at the reality of their situation. In looking at how things actually are, we can recognize what *is* true.

And it *is* true that:

- These are people who are not sure of who they are and who YOU are.
- These are people who do not remember.
- These are people who are confused.
- These are people who do not move easily because of their advanced age or various illnesses.
- They are dealing with pain.
- They can be difficult and challenging – life has become difficult and challenging for them.

But, despite all this, it is important to affirm the following:

- YES! They are highly intelligent and knowledgeable.
- YES! They know how to respect others and listen with that respect.
- YES! They need to express their feelings, because most of their communication with others involves practical issues: to make it through the day, week, month, hour. Everyone around them is certain these people are not connected to their emotions. On a day-to-day basis, who even has the strength or time to deal with feelings?
- And YES! They are capable of sharing, trusting, expressing their truth, enabling, giving, continuing and moving on – despite their disabilities and their sickness.

And . . .

- YES! They want to be stimulated.
- YES! We can create social cohesion within this group.
- YES! We can develop self-efficacy.
- YES! They are creative and spontaneous – Oh, yes – no problem there!
- And YES! Melabev is a happy place despite all the challenges our participants face daily.

Each session, the people in this group helped me to learn what they needed in order to function as a group, to participate and definitely improve their situation. I learned that through acting it out, *concretizing*, or through *role-playing*, *role reversals*, and *enactment*, they remembered. They internalized what they experienced in the sessions and some of it remained in their brains and so much of it stayed in their hearts.

In this group, it was very important to show the participants how much trust I had in their capabilities and competence. I was in their "yes" and they knew it. I learned from them, above all, that for people who have the misfortune to have any form of dementia, their routine lives are filled with negativity, humiliation and social isolation. This was a major issue that came up in a powerful session where I placed an *empty chair* in the center of our circle representing their families. This brought out many inner truths and their genuine pain could be heard loud and clear. In this particular session, one of the participants, addressing the empty chair, "said" to his son psychodramatically:

> You pass right over me. I can still do things. Maybe I can't remember, but I can hear. I have not lost all my abilities. And I still have a brain. You are talking about me right in front of me and it is humiliating to hear what you are saying.

This outpouring was emotionally echoed by others, as they took turns to speak to members of their families in the *empty chair*. We witnessed a strong sense of vitality, strength and will in the activity and in the *sharing*. They were not alone in their humiliating experiences; according to Tian Dayton (1994, p. 9), psychodrama lets us . . . "speak the words we dared not speak but have shouting within us".

Psychodrama lets us . . . "speak the words we dared not speak but have shouting within us".

It was also essential to empower them to trust in themselves. Moreover, the trust in the other group members was a major goal at the beginning of our journey. It became obvious that we were going to make it when 95-year-old Jacob (who mostly sat completely hunched over) said, at the end of our third session, "We need to be assured that what is said here remains confidential."

I saw then that they were warmed up for what J.L. Moreno called psychodrama, the "Theater of Truth". And when Jacob spoke now, his head was held up high with dignity. We could see his face – beaming with light and determination. I am sure that this experience and all of our interactive activities helped him maintain his dignity as a human being who is an active part of the community.

An Invitation to Meet Some of the Individuals

The first time I actually worked with the Challenge Group at Melabev I was moved to tears by their honesty. When, after a few sessions, we all stood in a line according to our age, we saw that the age span was very large. The group slowly grew and is still growing dynamically. The age range today spans from age 59 to age 100. I was not *close* to their age; I *was* their age. I was told by the staff that our Tuesday morning sessions were different from the rest of their time at the center. The people in our group were more awake, involved, vital, connected. And I had been under the impression that they were always so expressive.

I was told by the staff that our Tuesday morning sessions were different from the rest of their time at the center. The people in our group were more awake, involved, vital, connected. And I had been under the impression that they were always so expressive.

Let me introduce you to some of the people I have had the honor of working with since September 2015 and give you some general information about each of them. You will surely get to know them better through the description of the sessions. It is vital to understand the range of reasons for being in this group as well as the diversity of personalities. Not only were they from different backgrounds, most professional and some not, but the severity of their impairment was very dynamic, fluctuating and unpredictable. Even within each individual, there was a huge flux in the ebb and flow of their capabilities. From week to week, I might find the same person either better or worse. Here is a sampling from over 40 people who have participated in my five years of working in Melabev. Some have passed away or are no longer strong enough to come to the center or have been transferred to lower functioning groups. I was not involved in the intake for this group, so readers will in effect know as much about them as I did myself. In this introduction to our interactive process, I share my first impressions and the necessary information I received from the staff. To protect their privacy, I am not including information that will make the participants identifiable.

Adrienne: 84 years – she walked out ten minutes into her first meeting saying bitterly and with umbrage, "It's nobody's business how I am feeling!" However, a year later, after hearing about our sessions from her friends, she returned and became one of our star participants.

Avi: 65 years – had been a successful leading psychiatrist and was very interested in what could happen to him and the others in this circle of trust and action. In some sessions, he contributed major insights on our process. He was very aware of his deteriorating situation due to his Alzheimer's disease.

Barbara: 94 years – a very pleasant and sociable housewife, with a healthy need to talk. She was lonely and bored and was dealing with the normal issues of her age.

Benjy: 70 years – has Parkinson's disease and has lost significant memory unfortunately as a side effect of a new treatment. He was and, in many ways, still is a sharp businessman.

Brian: 91 years – a very dapper gentleman and successful business-man who is struggling to keep his dignity in his old age.

Carole: 92 years – almost blind and hard of hearing with deteriorating cognition but still able to express herself eloquently.

Daisy: 73 years – very lonely, chronically depressed and angry.

David: 93 years – a sweet, intelligent man. He could not see with his eyes, but he saw everything with his heart: gentleness, wisdom, depth and understanding. He had survived the Holocaust and he had become a famous watchmaker on the Upper East Side of Manhattan. Here I write more about him because he imme-diately had a huge impact on the group. He subtly let us know that customers like Gloria Swanson, Candice Bergen, Sidney Poitier, William Buckley and Arthur Rubenstein and many more had frequented his shop. His contributions to our sessions were precious and his death after one year with our group had a pro-found effect on us all! Once, he had even let us know that Gloria Swanson told him that his large earlobes signaled a long life.

Debra: 94 years – pain from various illnesses and difficulty in managing her hearing aid caused frustration and grouchiness. She could not remember anything. (She was the woman who was completely transformed when we did the Forest exercise mentioned above.)

Estelle: 72 years – very fragile, suffering from serious Parkinson's. Her hands shook all the time and it was extremely difficult for her to articulate her thoughts. She was always beautifully and fashionably dressed and accessorized.

Geoffrey: 87 years – a literature professor from one of the world's lead-ing universities. He was an expert on Shakespeare. He was very dignified and continually mentioned how difficult it was for him to have dementia.

Harvey: 89 years – widowed and lonely. He became acquainted with Melabev through accompanying his wife to the center for a number of years. After she passed away, he realized that the program would help him survive his aching loneliness and his increasing old age. His cognition level was quite high.

Jacob: 95 years – mentally as sharp as can be and brilliant. Before his retirement, he was an electrical engineer. Recently wid-owed, he was still mourning. He could not walk without assistance. He was so bent-over, I could not see his face. He had a tiny notebook and fancy pen in his shirt pocket to help him retain information that was important to him. He would constantly take them out and jot down whatever he needed to remember. Over time, he became the group voice on many issues. The group instinctively knew it was worth waiting for him to raise his head slowly, collect his thoughts and then share his words of wisdom.

Lila: 80 years – was a social worker. She was very aware of her progressing Alzheimer's disease. When I bumped into her one evening in a local restaurant, she said, "I know I've met you and I know I really like you. But I don't know where I know you from. Can you remind me how I know you?"

Lilly: 94 years – had lived in India, London and finally, Israel. She was the matriarch of a large, wonderful family. No matter what we did, she was always successful in coming up with an appropriate quote from Omar Khayyam to summarize the session. Paradoxically, every time I walked into the room she would ask her neighbor: "Who is this lady?"

Lionel: 73 years – extremely creative and talented. He was cheerful, but that covered up severe pain, frustration and anger. He had many health issues, including diabetes. It became obvious that role-playing was a healthy form of venting his feelings.

Martin: 88 years – Was a sports teacher and a successfully recognized basketball coach. His progressing Alzheimer's disease did not affect his friendliness and his need to socialize.

Moe: 95 years – The oldest participant in our group. Worked as a municipal employee. He came to Melabev with the sole purpose of getting out to socialize. He has no dementia but his age has slowed him down. None of his children live in Israel but he speaks to them very often. There is much about his sweet manner and kind disposition in PART V of this book where his 100th Zoom birthday party is described in detail. His contributions were filled with charm and honesty.

Monica: 90 years – had been a curator in one of the world's most prestigious art museums. Her Alzheimer's disease was emotionally painful. Her exciting past and her ability to articulate clearly and easily despite the disease made her an important contributor to the flow of our sessions.

Moshe: 87 years – repeatedly fell asleep but loved being connected to other people who understood his situation.

Herbie: 68 years – was afraid to speak. Eventually, he participated honestly and courageously. Others in the group consistently encouraged him and empowered him with their responses to his honest, sincere and witty responses. He had early onset Alzheimer's disease.

Robert: 59 years – much younger than everyone else, but unfortunately suffering from early onset Alzheimer's disease. His wife brings him to the Melabev center just for psychodrama and music to try to stimulate him after she has been coping alone with him for six years.

Rosie: 88 years – totally paralyzed. She was confined to an elaborate wheel chair and had difficulty projecting her voice. She could not breathe without her oxygen tank.

Simmy: 91 years – he was always smiling and he didn't know why. This man had been a brilliant, world-renowned psychologist.

Therapeutic Goals of Group Work

This was a group of people who were struggling with the greatest loss of all: their memories, their cognition, their physical and cognitive function, and their dignity. In short, their very selves.

> This was a group of people who were struggling with the greatest loss of all: their memories, their cognition, their physical and cognitive function, their dignity. In short, their very selves.

I felt privileged to be working with people who needed to surface out of their pit of dementia and find recognition; people with rich and varied backgrounds, high intelligence and heart-warming charm. These people possessed both culture and dynamic pasts. When I decided to work with them, I made the following decisions that governed my approach:

- To believe in them and help them believe in themselves.
- To respect them and their situation.
- To never go below their level, but rather, to challenge them to use their experience, wisdom and intelligence.
- To be empathic.
- To be flexible and spontaneous.
- To use humor and be playful and light.
- Do *with* instead of *to*.
- Always be open and honest with them and trust the truth, because psychodrama is the "theater of truth".

In truth, all these decisions are interconnected, and each one flows on naturally from the previous one, so if we believe in these special people, we will respect them, and so on.

After working with my Melabev Group, I deeply understood that my list of goals must expand. I must also help them:

- Build trust in themselves, in the group, in the process and in the staff.
- Address their social isolation; their loneliness, boredom, depression and helplessness.
- Validate their feelings and help them to realize that they are not alone and they are understood.

- Help them validate one another through our experiential work.
- Create an environment where they would feel safe and secure.
- Help them be in their "YES".
- Help them feel connected.
- Facilitate a supportive environment for them to express their potential.
- Understand, accept and flow with the fact that, because of the age and fragility of the participants, this group would have a sizable turnover.
- Find ways for them to retrieve memories through experiential expressive work; *role reversals, concretizing, mirroring, scene settings*, imaginary photos, associations, drama games, improvisations – in one word, *DOING!!!*
- Give them something to look forward to.

And YES, as we developed into a fully functioning psychodrama group, my list of goals expanded exponentially. Some five years later, we have a dynamic group of sixteen to twenty-two senior citizens aged 59–100 who come alive every Tuesday morning through experiential validation.

Some five years later, we have a dynamic group of sixteen to twenty-two senior citizens aged 59–100 who come alive every Tuesday morning through experiential validation.

The members of my group share their life experiences, problems, frustrations, conflicts, insights and their feelings! They now share all of this with confidence, trust and sincere, deep compassion.

These wonderful people, with their vast range of abilities and disabilities, are active participants in a group. They are empowered through sharing and showing. They do not feel useless. In fact, the group has such a special "vibe" that all the volunteers and staff at this day-center love to join in with them, and they relish witnessing the magic in our circle.

How did we accomplish this?
What did we do?
What tools of psychodrama were used successfully?
How was this group accommodated with its special needs and limitations?

I would love to continue here with our process but, for the readers who are unfamiliar with psychodrama, I will add an introduction to psychodrama so that as you go on, you will be better informed.

What Is Psychodrama? Why Is It Good for This Population?

Now that you are acquainted with the people in this group and my professional background, goals and attitude, I would like to take you through the entire process, with this group as the example. I would like to equip you with a brief introduction to psychodrama and how it can benefit these people.

What is therapeutic for this population? It is a well-known fact that music is therapeutic and even magical for people with dementia. Music is in fact the most popular activity at the Melabev Center, especially with the lowest functioning group. The participants sing along and are happy to be in a rhythm together. No one talks about themselves or how they are feeling. There is no interaction per se and no spontaneity, but there is definitely a retrieval of lyrics and melodies accompanied by memories and a positive energy. It's only good!

However, the music sessions can be seen as mostly passive because the participants do not have to initiate anything. On the other hand, psychodrama requires active participation from everyone in the group.

It turns out that the process of building a psychodrama group proved to be a most viable tool for the people in my group. Unlike music, group psychodrama is a type of *experiential* action-based therapy in which people explore issues and conflicts by acting out events and situations. By *doing* and interacting in a group setting, the participants learn about themselves through role-playing and role-reversals, mirroring, sociometric exercises, empathic doubles and sharing how they feel. The participants gain greater understanding and insight into their lives and experiences, resolve issues, and practice new life skills and behaviors.

I will explain these techniques with examples from our sessions in My Psychodrama Tool Box in PART III and in all of PART IV. Readers who want a more scientific approach to spontaneity and psychodrama should read the article listed in the bibliography by Dani Yaniv. The following is a quote from that article.

> Psychodrama uses a dramatic theatrical format to allow clients to enact emotions, experiences and meaningful events in life, thus turning the abstract into concrete. Through dramatic action, the client explores an internal world, reaching insights about self and others, experiences what could never happen, and develops better living skills. Based on action and the enhancement of spontaneity and creativity, psychodrama assists clients in facing life challenges, examine alternative solutions, and sometimes adapt to their situation with peaceful acceptance. The protagonist in psychodrama is invited to actually become the "thing" that s/he is referring to, be it a person or an abstract concept, like passion.

J. L. Moreno's following three phrases form the basis of my group psychodrama work, and are repeatedly mentioned in this book: "Psychodrama is the theatre of truth", "Don't tell me, show me" and "Trust the process". They are the secret ingredients of our success.

What was this success? This entire procedure wove an intimate connection between the members. They began to understand that their truth was interesting to others. The authentic expression that evolves from a psychodrama session initiated a change in attitude, feelings, and affected their understanding and functioning and the ability to socialize. As the participants began to trust the process, trust the leader, trust one another and ultimately, and most importantly, trust themselves within an interactive group – they came alive. They rediscovered their identity with pride.

Two basic components of psychodrama are spontaneity and creativity. The participants discovered that they had the courage to respond spontaneously without giving it a thought. Before they knew it, they were totally engrossed within interactive activities. They were enjoying every minute and looked forward to the next session. The saying, "memory brings identity" in this situation also seemed to work the other way around, with identity leading to memory. Information was being retrieved and shared. By listening to one another, they were learning about themselves. You will see examples of uninhibited statements in role-playing that elicited sincere and brave sharing. This resulted in the empowering of each individual through deep and creative interaction.

In psychodrama, we bypass cognition as we know it. We use action, doing, showing, spontaneity and creativity as the stimulus for interaction. We validate authentic expression and the retrieval of language, memories from the past and even short-term memories. Something happens to the participants that triggers brain waves that have been dormant. This *doing* brings a new energy to the participants, expands their options by discovering new routes and new pathways that free the participants from restraints. In my opinion, for this population, *doing* leads to being. An essential goal in my work is to bypass the stuck place through incentives that trigger spontaneous interaction.

I was encouraged to try to release the inner world, imprisoned in our participants, through action, creativity and spontaneity in the techniques of psychodrama. One of my mentors was Dr. Adam Blatner (1937–2021), a child and adult psychiatrist and a leading psychodramatist. His book, Acting-In, was very helpful to me in my instinctive work with all the populations I have worked with and especially with people suffering from old age and dementia in all its forms. I hope this long quote will encourage you to read on and find the magic of connecting through the action method called psychodrama. Dr. Blatner said memorably:

Many of the most powerful active approaches in contemporary psychotherapy and education are derived from the method of psychodrama, in which a person is helped to imagine and enact a problem instead of just talking about it. Psychodrama and its associated methods of sociodrama, role playing, and sociometry were invented around the 1930s by Jacob L. Moreno, M.D. (1889–1974).

The psychodramatic method integrates the modes of cognitive analysis with the dimensions of experiential and participatory involvement. Actually "doing" the interaction, engaging one's own physical body and imagination as if the situation were unfolding in the present moment, brings into consciousness a host of ideas and feelings not generally accessed through simply talking about the situation. The non-verbal elements of communication not only act interpersonally, but also as inner cues, so that, for example, behaving in a more angry or frightened manner will evoke an awareness of emotions which may have been otherwise, repressed.

Action approaches are especially useful in therapy not only with patients who have little capacity for intellectual and verbal exploration. . . .

One of psychodrama's most significant advantages is that it converts the participant's urge towards "acting-out" into the more constructive channel of "acting-in".

(Blatner, 1996, XII)

And now what was *our* process? Read on and enjoy.
    What was *my* Process?

    I'll begin at the beginning.

Part II

Initiating the Process

Starting a New Group

Meeting the Group and Meeting Myself

The Melabev Center had decided to offer the Challenge Group one more day in the weekly schedule. It was the brainstorm of Jennie, one of their leaders, to find someone who could help this group express their feelings through drama. Before actually starting to work with them, we had a short introductory session in order to get acquainted with the members of our group and the staff. I met their great Tuesday leaders: Jennie and Howie. Jennie's wisdom, devotion and caring were evident all the time; and Howie's humor, personality and talent were always helpful. It was obvious to me that this Group loved their leaders. They always knew just what to say to each person.

I also met a circle of people who were non-responsive, apathetic and very resistant to trying something new. And they met a gray-haired woman with two bags filled with scarves who was trying too hard and too fast to win them over.

Then came our first official session. I will never forget that Tuesday morning in October 2015. Today would be their first drama session. As you can imagine, I was nervous and unsure but also determined to try my best. Somehow, I managed to transmute my anxiety into positive energy. (I have become pretty good at doing that over the years.) I take my place at the head of the circle. The members of this group have no idea what I am about to do with them. Their comments are *not* funny. This is what I am hearing from all over, "Oy, the lady with the schmattes (rags) is here."

"What does she want from us??"
"What is Drama anyway!?"
"I never liked that kind of stuff."

Yes, that introductory getting acquainted meeting definitely did NOT work. Fortunately, I have a few exercises for an opening session that are

DOI: 10.4324/9781003321705-2

comfortable, non-threatening and just what we all need – simple, novel ways to get acquainted.

I know from experience and many past challenges that these exercises work with every group that needs the incentive to open up, get started and connect. My enthusiasm helps me overcome their resistance to trying something new and unfamiliar, even though, somewhere inside of me, I am feeling like "the *schmatte* lady".

Creating a Circle of Trust

I sit in my seat at the head of the circle. I am both inspired and humbled by their need. I explain that *DRAM* in Greek means – *to enact or to do by action*. This is enough explanation for now. I tell them that in our sessions by *doing* and *enacting* we will learn more about ourselves and one another and have fun at the same time. Because they are listening to me attentively, I have the feeling that they actually believe me. We are on our way. I begin with my instructions.

"Say your name and add an adjective that describes you."

I give them examples and options such as: "I am spontaneous Tzippi." "I am hyperactive Tzippi." "I am sensitive or empathic Tzippi." "I am creative Tzippi." This is a sneaky way to tell them something about myself and to invite them to do the same. They do.

The person to the right will repeat what was said (for some people, this is a major accomplishment). She or he then announces her or his name along with a descriptive adjective. "This is spontaneous Tzippi and I am friendly Martin." The person to his or her right will repeat what Martin said and add his name with a descriptive adjective. "This is friendly Martin and I am caring Pauline." In my other groups, I would have them repeat three or four; for this group, one repeat is enough. Everyone hears their name and connects to their personal identity.

Up to now, we've had audio mirroring. I now add a *DOING*. Whenever something significant is said, the rest of the group raises their right hand from zero on their knee, to ten – as high as they can go – to *show* how much they identify with what was said. In psychodrama, this is called a *spectrogram*, a word which reminds me of graphs and other enemies. I prefer the term *sociometrics* – and that's what I have used in all my courses, workshops, and my sessions with this group. Most of the participants cannot walk independently, so they show us where they stand by raising their hand. They do not have to leave their chair.

For example, "My name is Adele, and, I am . . . caring."

Everyone in the group raises their hand from zero to ten to show how caring they are. This ritual has become natural to them. By showing, they are sharing, identifying with one another and collecting options. I like to tell my groups to listen with a "third ear". This is the ear that internalizes what someone in the group has said and strengthens our self-awareness. These are some of the adjectives they have used to describe themselves over these five years: loyal, thankful, optimistic, witty, witchy, thoughtful, enthusiastic, self-contained, happy, mischievous, cheerful, shy, active, morose, good-natured, friendly, funny, energetic, adventurous, practical, pensive, sarcastic, sensitive, imaginative, creative, outgoing, one of a kind, helpful, leader, teachable, indulgent, assertive, half-deaf, loveable, moody, selfish, zany, curious, musical, grateful to be alive.

These descriptions have become options for them to add to their own self-image to strengthen their identity and a means of identifying with others in the group. The sociometric spectrogram validates their self-perception. I would always suggest that they listen with ears that connect, and apply to themselves and that they ask themselves: who has a trait that I also have? Who has a trait that I need? I must admit, I was doing this too! This exercise facilitates a form of mirroring – both visual and audio. More important, their trust in me, and the process, took a giant leap forward. They were with me – what a relief!

Actually, every time someone new would join our group, I would repeat this exercise. The participants would never tire of it and it is a way to measure cognitive development. Each time the participants would give a more sophisticated adjective to portray their essence. I suppose I should evaluate this information but, as you will see by reading further, I would rather *do* than analyze and measure.

Another exercise that requires eye contact and connecting is to have them simply announce their names from wherever they are sitting . . . in alphabetical order. They might need help from the leader with a statement like, "Let's see who is next. We had Annette for the letter A and Barbara, for B. Anyone here whose name starts with C? What about D? Dave that's you." Dave will definitely become alert and announce his name as everyone looks around the room to see who is next. This is another way to be certain that everyone in the circle participates and has the feeling of being an integral part of a group. By simply announcing their names, they are asserting themselves in a primary way.

Summary of Practical Applications

- Give your group examples so that they are sure of the directions.
- Saying and hearing our name and the names of others in the group is so simple and yet extremely important.
- Ask the participants to find an adjective that describes them.
- Remind them to listen with a "third ear" that will hear options, opportunities to identify with others, and validations.
- Spectrograms can be done from their seats by raising their hands from 0 to 10.
- Encourage eye contact with exercises that require looking around at everyone in the circle.
- Many exercises encourage full participation.

Following Session: Developing Cohesion in the Group

This time I walk in feeling so much more comfortable with my group and with myself. They are already eager to discover what we will be doing today. I am no longer the *schmatte lady*. Actually, some of them have no idea who I am but they quickly remember when I pull an object out of my drama basket. This also reminds me of who I am!

I take out a soft, square lap-sized pillow. The task is to pass or throw the pillow to someone about whom you would like to know more. I know that Martin was once a champion basketball player and I say:

> I can't wait to see how Martin passes the pillow. Actually, this exercise is supposed to be done with a ball, but . . . if we don't catch the ball, we will be very busy finding it. If we don't catch the pillow, it will just nestle on the floor. And we can try again.

Yes, I am a part of this, and all of our exercises as is the rest of the staff. Our participation is essential. Our energy is contagious.

To continue with the directions, I explain that we hold the pillow on our lap with two hands. We describe the person we have chosen by telling the group what that person is wearing in a way that he or she will know it is definitely them and no one else in the group. We find something unique in the person's attire. I demonstrate "I am throwing the pillow to a woman wearing a navy-blue skirt and a pink blouse. Her jewelry consists of a pearl necklace, gold earrings with a ruby stone and a gold watch. She has New Balance sneakers on her feet and short white socks". Barbara, who is seated to the right of me, immediately knows it is definitely her. I wish you could see the gleam of recognition in her eyes when I add, "and her name is___" and she proudly announces her name. I throw the pillow to her and she catches it with relative ease. I then ask my question, "How many children, grandchildren or great-grandchildren do you have?"

A simple non-mathematical question that does not tax their cognition, such as "What's your favorite food?" "Are your shoes comfortable?" works here.

Now Barbara is certain of what she should do. But, to make it easier, the instructions are to describe and then throw the pillow to someone from the first person on my left on the other side of the circle, to the fifth. Let's say, from Martin to Pauline. This way everyone's eyes are focused on that section of the circle and it is easier for Barbara to make her selection from this limited group.

It always drove me crazy when the kindergarten teacher would say to a child who is celebrating his birthday in the kindergarten, "Pick someone to give you a birthday blessing." This hapless 5-year-old participant has a serious dilemma. He has to choose one – only one. He knows that if he doesn't pick the bully, he is in trouble. If he picks a girl, they might laugh at him and he must pick his mother's best friend's son and what about the kids in his carpool, or maybe his cousin!? So, he is by now in a state of utter confusion. Too much pressure on one 5-year-old participant! There is no way he is going to be able to decide calmly and with assurance. It is much more effective to limit the choices. This is true for children – of all ages, even 95!

Back to our group. Barbara throws the pillow to Herbie who is the only one in the room and certainly in his small group of five, who is wearing a baseball cap and has bright yellow socks. Barbara winds up her arm and joyfully throws the pillow to Herbie . . . and so on. . . . In this way, everyone receives a moment of what Kohut calls *grandiosity* (See Chapter on Kohut in PART III). That person gets all the attention for a few seconds. You can see it in the light in their face, the way they hold their heads up high and smile. In addition, everyone has to connect to someone else in the room, via the pillow and the description. We learn classification. We are beginning to realize that we are not alone. We are part of a group. There is a lot of eye contact and everyone opens their mouth and speaks. We are again reminded of their names and, through the questions, we learn something about them. And, of course, they get to throw this pillow and catch it. So simple. So important. And I get the ACTION and INTERACTION that I so love!

Everyone receives a moment of what Kohut calls *grandiosity*.

Summary of Practical Applications

- Throwing a soft pillow in order to connect.
- When asking a member to throw the soft pillow to someone in the group, minimize the choices to help that person focus in.
- Tell that person to describe who has been chosen by telling the group what that person is wearing in a way that he or she will know it is definitely them and no one else in the group. And, once again, the participants get to announce their names.

Warm-ups

I have come to realize that we all need and have our individual ways of warming up before beginning to work on something. Before I start anything, even cooking, I need a perfect cup of coffee. (Yes, that makes for a lot of caffeine!) As a psychodrama facilitator, I need a warm-up exercise that gets me started as well as the group. A warm-up is an activity that triggers involvement, creates cohesion within the group and invites follow-up. Sometimes, a simple ritual like bringing in different puppets each time as a metaphor to what I want to accomplish with the group through psychodrama in the specific meeting, opens the session and is an invitation for more. (See the section called "Creating a New Group Between Lockdowns" in PART VII.)

The following sections show a variety of warm-ups to get the group involved and ready for action. They are a stimulus and a relaxant at the same time. I need them as much as the group! They help build a circle of trust, safety and possibility and arouse our spontaneity.

I am going to start with an example of a technique used for a warm-up that I use very often because it always works for me.

Concretizing: The Language of Scarves

This section is proportionately large because I used this technique very often at the beginning of our process to give expression to the inner world of the participants. There is a form of *embodiment* and *projection* here that is basic in drama therapy – according to Sue Jennings, one of the foremost practitioners, teachers, and authors in the field of drama therapy, in her two books, 1973 and 1987 (see Bibliography).

Multi-colored scarves are spread out on a table at the head of the group circle. The opportunity to play with these soft, colorful pieces of material and use them to symbolize abstract things is a good way to begin a process with this population. The softness and flexibility of the scarves provide sensory stimulation and primary pleasure (Images 2.1–2.3).

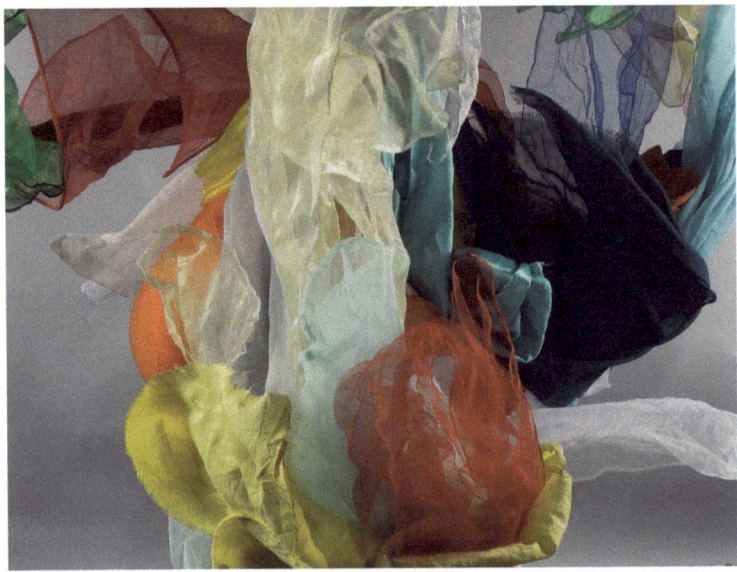

Image 2.1

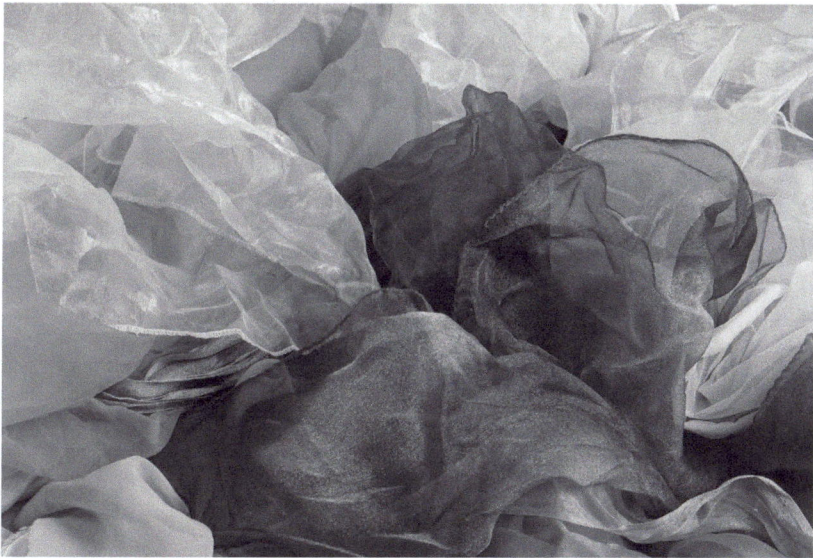

Image 2.2

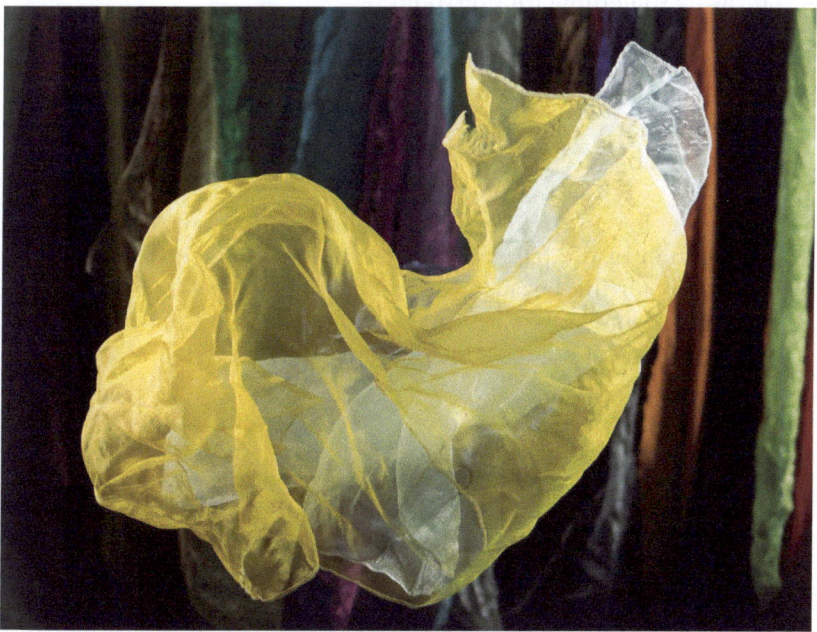

Image 2.3 Concretizing with multi-colored scarves

Furthermore, the use of scarves of different sizes and varied shades of colors is used to *concretize*. By this, I mean that we can SEE what is being expressed and developed and create a situation where we all witness and DO. As a result, we are better able to integrate and REMEMBER.

Here are some of the concretizing exercises:

I ask the participants:

What is Melabev (the Jerusalem Day-Care Center where our meetings regularly take place) for you? Pick a colored scarf that symbolizes what you want to say. We will place them on the floor, in the center and sculpt what Melabev is for you.

These are some of the responses to my question:

- Gold = hope
- Royal blue = caring
- Green = growth
- Aqua = flowing
- Navy blue = almost like a prison
- A few bright colors = cheerful
- Orange = exposure to other people
- Brown = something for everyone

The *concretization* and the ability to SEE, helps them understand, express and internalize.

We use the scarves, as a warm-up to see and concretize many subjects. The instructions are:

Find a color and texture that symbolizes a word, association or description of the particular subject. The language of the colored scarves is terrific because you are never wrong. Once you pick a scarf, it is what YOU want to say by showing. With the scarves, let's sculpt with a color and shape that best depicts you.

I continue:

If we were creating a work of modern art on this wall and everyone here is represented by a different color and shape, what color would you pick to personify you? You decide on a color. Your personal decision is always correct. It is the way you see yourself in color. Every color can mean something else to different people. That's fine. Have fun with the colors! Look at these scarves and connect to one color that you feel represents you.

This is a concrete personification, and hence the term *concretization.*

These exercises are person-centered where the person knows he or she is an integral part of a group. The individual expression creates something new and dynamic as you will see in the development of this exercise with the scarves.

I continue further:

> Now, let's sculpt Our Group. Tell us all where to place the scarf you selected so that we can *see* you as part of the group. (It is necessary to give this instruction because some members of the group are incapable to getting up and doing it themselves) Now, we can see this group. This is our group. What do we see here? Are you happy with the way you are depicted here? Would you like to move to the center? Would you rather be on the periphery? Are you too big? Too small? What would you like to change?

The important message here is that each individual participant is an integral part of a group.

This is a very powerful exercise in group dynamics. Through the use of the scarves, the participants are able to see themselves as an integral part of a whole. At the same time, these exercises with the scarves expand our knowledge of the abstract functionalism of the people in our Challenged Group. The staff is able to observe our participants functioning on a higher level of cognition through the facilitation of abstract thinking, thanks to the tool of concretizing with the scarves. The fact that most of the members – not all – can do this is significant in evaluating the cognition level of the people in our group.

Following is a selection of subjects that can be concretized with scarves.

- A group contract: Letting the colors represent rules for our sessions, like not interrupting, respecting the privacy of everyone in the group. What is said in this room – stays in this room! No phones, no private conversations, no judging.
- Sculpting roles in our lives. Instructions: Let's sculpt the ideal: parent, grandparent, sibling, friend, or patient (Image 2.4).
- A birthday gift to Israel or to any country.
- A birthday gift to someone in the group who is celebrating a birthday.

We give that person the scarves that symbolize our greetings and gifts. The birthday person ends up being draped in beautiful, meaningful scarves. The embodiment here is almost primary!

- I address the Group and say: "Today, my mood is cheerful . . . (grumpy, tired, curious, excited, nervous, frightened, concerned,

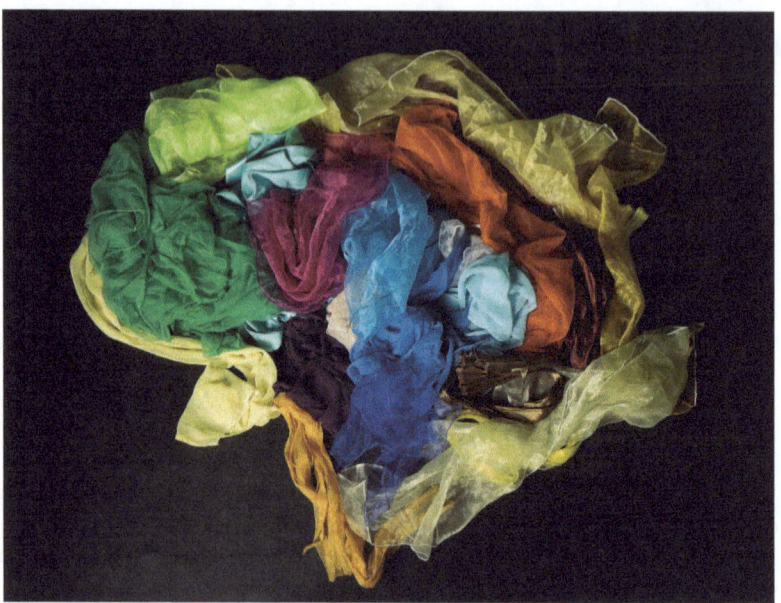

Image 2.4 Let's sculpt a sibling

waiting, concerned, anticipating, vital, positive, thankful, alive . . .). Assign a color to this mood and pick a scarf to match."

Concretizing with the different colors in the scarves enables us to identify with others, to receive validation of our own feelings and to gain new options for our volatile moods.

Here's another exercise that I will describe in detail in order to illustrate how the scarves technique can develop into a rich, revealing, therapeutic session.

A Descriptive Session: Sculpting an Ideal Leader

The setting for this session was a Tuesday which also happened to be Election Day for the United States President. Events such as this can provide an excellent trigger for concretizing exercises.

Instructions: Let's sculpt an ideal leader of a country. (They all agree with me that it would be incredibly wonderful if we could only do this. And they know!) We will use the colored scarves so that we can see this ideal leader.

Everyone is asked to think of essential traits of an ideal leader. I repeat, "The beauty of the use of scarves for illustrating is that whatever choices are made, they are correct." Everyone participates and connects by simply selecting a scarf. I ask them for the word they wish to choose, and the color that symbolizes that word (for them). They consider it and it usually takes a little while as they look over the heap of colors. When they choose a color – let's say red – I then gather up all the hues of red: flaming, scarlet, cherry red, blood red, brick red, apple red, blush red, rose red, crimson red, scarlet red . . . The scarves also have different textures and sizes. I bring this sampling of red scarves and ask them to touch them and deeply consider which scarf is exactly right for their word. Watching their process of deciding which scarf and which hue of the color shows us how significant and therapeutic this form of concretizing is and strengthens the therapeutic value of color.

Those who can walk on their own get up, walk to the heap of scarves on the table, choose one and place it in our sculpture. However, instead of getting up themselves, 90% of the group tell a volunteer where to place the scarf. Everyone gets a chance to hold their scarf and enjoy the sense of touch and define the color they have chosen and we begin. This is a dynamic process. Someone starts as a trigger. Many times, it is necessary for the leader to pave the way and illustrate this new form of abstract expression with a few examples. They very quickly learn the language of the scarves and use the colors to express their ideas and feelings. I must admit that not all of our participants are capable of abstract thinking, but, somehow, they catch on or simply pick a color that they love. This, too, is therapy! And there is always the challenge from the three members who call these scarves "Tzippi's *schmattes* (rags)".

Here is an example of colors chosen to illustrate the qualities of an ideal leader. The members contributed to the creation of a scarf sculpture. It was a group creation. They each experienced the pride of group work and the sense of being a part of something bigger than each individual.

- White = honesty
- Gray = intelligence
- Royal blue = brave
- True blue = truthful
- Purple = keeps promises and decisions
- Green = integrity
- Darker green = comfortably wealthy and financially independent
- Blue and White = patriotic
- Bright Yellow = aware
- Orange= cooperative
- Gold = confident
- Silver = dignity
- White = healthy
- Navy Blue = wise
- Orange = peaceful

- Light Blue = level-headed
- Brown = experienced
- Magenta = cultured
- Purple = unflappable
- Rainbow = charismatic
- Pale Pink = has humility
- Gray = pretty accepting
- Transparent white = transparent
- Pale Blue = fair-minded
- Black = not perfect

The next step is to ask them to think about:

- What do you have in common with this ideal leader?
- What can you take from this ideal leader?

After they think about this and check how many of those characteristics they have in common with our sculptured ideal leader, they realize that, as heads of their families, they too are leaders.

Then they are asked: What traits do you have that you could give to this ideal leader? Here are a few of their responses:

- Red = sense of humor
- Purple = trustworthy
- Green = respectful
- Navy blue = educated
- Black = not perfect

And a few more exercises where the scarves help give expression:

After any traumatic event, such as a fire, plane crash or terror attack, it is essential to process the shock and fear. Ask the participants to pick a scarf that expresses what each person needs right now. Tell them to pick a color and give it a word such as "aqua" – to relax, "pink" – a hug. We then sculpt our "support sculpture" with the various scarves and continue spontaneously.

For personal and group feedback: pick a scarf with the color that expresses – What came up in this session that I want or need to take? What came up in this session that I want to leave or throw away?

This is an effective way to summarize the session and give personal and group feedback.

After these subjects are illustrated, in front of them, through concretizing with the scarves, mostly as a warm-up, open the subject to share feelings, thoughts and experiences connected to this subject. We "speak" to a grandchild, sibling, friend, doctor or neighbor (addressing them as if they were right here) through *role reversal* or by talking to the *empty chair* or we hear what they want to say to us from the *empty chair.*

So many of my students, over the years, have purchased arrays of scarves to use in their work. The art therapists that I worked with especially appreciated the flexibility and simplicity of expression through the use of scarves. For the life of me I cannot draw and the scarves always painted the perfect picture for me.

Opening With a Sentence

We have seen that the scarves work as a warm-up for various subjects. Another technique that can be used for warm-up, using triggers to entice each individual to participate to bring out what they have inside them is to open with a sentence. This can be so much fun. Almost every sentence works.

- When I need to cope, I . . .
- I am independent when . . . (Independence Day)
- I need help with . . .
- I am dependent when . . .
- I need to ask for help when . . .
- I moved to Israel because . . .
- I moved to Israel because . . .
- Why did I . . . ?
- When I'm upset, I . . .
- When I feel lonely, I . . .
- I feel relaxed when . . .
- I am defiant, determined, when . . .
- I am sorry that . . .
- A hero is . . .
- I am a hero when . . .
- A gift I would like to receive is . . .
- A subject/issue, I would like to work on is . . . .
- I am thankful for . . . (Thanksgiving holiday)
- Happiness is . . . (Purim holiday)
- It is *after the Holidays.* I am now going to . . . .
- I have . . .
- I need . . .
- I want . . .
- I should . . .
- I can choose . . .
- I can . . .
- I can't . . . .

For example:

> "I can . . .
> I can admit I can't remember everyone's name.
> I can play the piano without looking.
> I can type without looking.
> (I could see their eyes lighting up as they each thought of something to share with the group-every one!)
> I can make people laugh.
> I can swim.
> I can cook.
> I can paint.
> I can think of happy times.
> I can read Hebrew, play the trombone, dance, belly dance, and lecture.
> (She was *sooo* empowered)
> I can read Russian.
> I can memorize poetry.
> I can read.
> I can plan my day.
> I can smile.
> I can style hair.
> I can appreciate my son.
> I can come to Melabev.
> I can appreciate other people.

Empowering Subjects as Incentives to Connecting

A lot of sessions begin with the introduction of a subject as a warm-up. Start by saying today our subject is . . .

Many times, simply announcing a subject is actually a warm-up. A simple sentence leads to connecting, sharing and reflective thinking. It triggers them. Some of these sessions that evoke interesting and sensitive responsiveness appear in detail in the Appendix.

- What is the light in your life?
- How do *you* light up the world?
- What do *you do* to bring light into your life?
- What is the message that you pass down to your children and grandchildren? What is your credo? (your *vehigadita le bincha* as written in the Passover Haggadah)
- What have you done in the past year to improve the quality of your life?
- How do you cope?
- How do you help other people?
- Remember a good deed that someone did for you.

- Remember a good deed that you did for someone else.
- Remember a special gift that you gave to someone.
- Remember a special gift that someone gave to you.
- What calms you down when you are very anxious?
- A decision that you can make for yourself?
- What do *you* need from these sessions?

What do *you* need from these sessions?

- Let your shoes tell us what steps you have taken this year to make your life better.
- Let's recall special moments in history, in your lifetime, that you remember.
- What does the word "reading" make you think of?
- A conflict or issue you would like to work on.
- Advice to your children or grandchildren when there is a change in their life.
- What does the word "cousin" bring up for you?
- What is your association with the word – LOVE?
- From the *Wizard of Oz*: What is "HOME" for you?
- What would you ask the Wizard to give you?
- How does the word "routine" make you feel?
- What do you take for granted?
- Tell us of a time when you met a challenge successfully.
- A gift that you received from your mother.
- A gift that you received from your father.

These are all subjects that evoke a quick and easy response. This helps the members retrieve their words. Listening to others encourages the participants to speak up and experience being an integral part of a discussion. Many of these people had given up hope of ever participating in the types of interactions we are having.

Many of these people had given up hope of ever participating in the types of interactions we are having.

Their families would report to the Center that they loved to talk about what we did in the Tuesday morning psychodrama sessions. The rationale of involvement, expression and language development *is* indeed empowering.

Using Personal Experience to Encourage Participation

Many of the subjects brought up, come from my life experiences and from the here and now, and serve as genuine invitations for members of the Group to join in, warm up and express themselves comfortably. These subjects reflect daily personal experiences. The participants feel comfortable expressing themselves in front of everyone else because they are able to identify with the material. The fact that the subjects are close to their daily reality makes it easier for them to formulate words and sentences and in so doing, express themselves with confidence and authority.

- "Today is my birthday – let's work on memories of birthday presents that we received and cherished."
- "This morning, I caught my finger in the door. The pain was unbearable. Even though I was alone, I cried. What do *you* do when you're in pain?"
- "My brother is visiting me. Let's work on the subject of siblings."
- "I lost my favorite earring. I can't forgive myself."
- "My family surprised me with a birthday party. I am overwhelmed."
- "I just started cleaning my home for Passover. When we clean for Passover, we do a lot of inventory. Let's clean our personal world for Passover and first take an inventory of our lives and see what we have. I have. . . ."
- Now that the cleaning for Passover is done, let's see what we want to throw away.

One member said, "I have nothing to throw away." Another member replied, "Then you must be kosher for Passover." This humor surfaced as this fairly new member began to trust himself and enjoy poking innocent fun at someone in the group.

After you try some of these warm-up exercises, I am sure you will discover and then agree with Marcia Karp that:

> The warm-up serves to produce an atmosphere of creative possibility. The first phase weaves a basket of safety in which the individual can begin to trust the director, the group and the method. When the room has its arms around you, it is possible to be that which you thought you couldn't, to express that which seemed impossible to express.
>
> Karp, 1998, *An Introduction to Psychodrama* (p. 3)

Summary of Practical Applications

- It is important to engage the participants in a natural way that will lead to honest expression, social cohesion, and self-efficacy via psychodrama.

- Use warm-ups as triggers to action and interaction.
- Scarves of all colors, puppets, playmobile and simple household items help the members concretize and *see* what they have been expressing. pressing
- Simple sentences, an interesting or personal comment or story stimulate participation.
- Almost any familiar subject can warm up your group and encourage them to connect.
- The transparency of the leader, when bringing a personal relevant story, encourages free, open expression.

Part III

Techniques and Tools

My Psychodrama Tool Box

I would really like to continue with the action part but I feel that first I should open my psychodrama toolbox and give those of you who have no idea what psychodrama is some background information and how psychodrama could be applied to this population.

Jacob Levy Moreno, the father of psychodrama, was born in Bucharest, Romania, on May 18, 1889, and died in Beacon, New York on May 14, 1974. He always said, "Don't tell me – show me." Following here are the tools of psychodrama that I was able to adapt to the level of this group. My goals were to give the participants ways to show, see and then share.

If you need a more detailed explanation of this method and these terms, see the section on *psychodrama* and use the Glossary. Throughout the book, I will bring numerous examples of all of these terms and techniques. The terms will be italicized throughout to aid understanding. Robert Landy summarizes terms of psychodrama so succinctly for his readers on role theory in Drama Therapy in his book, when he explains the essence of psychodrama, that I will quote directly from him here:

> Moreno's theory of role is an active and interactive one. The personality is developed as one plays out the many possibilities of being. These possibilities include playing real or ideal roles of *protagonist, auxiliary ego, double and director.* The *protagonist* is the central figure in the psychodrama. *Auxiliary egos* are antagonists or those who challenge or support the *protagonist.* The *double* is an alter ego representing the inner thoughts and feelings of the *protagonist* and *auxiliary egos.* And the director is the leader of the psychodrama who moves the other players in and out of role and generally attempts to explore and resolve a protagonist's dilemma.
>
> (Robert Landy, Persona and Performance: The Meaning
> of Role in Theater Therapy and Everyday Life,
> New York: Guilford, 1993, p. 24)

DOI: 10.4324/9781003321705-3

From the beginning, *Doubles* were used whenever possible. A double says what someone is feeling but is not saying. The doubles will be printed in a lighter shade throughout the book to signify that they are not spoken by the person. *My double for you, the reader who is not a therapist, could possibly be: I don't know anything about psychodrama. How will I be able to understand? I really need this book!* As a result of this double, I will bring a brief explanation here, as a starter, and I will elaborate and explain very clearly throughout the book.

We carried out *enactments* by staging scenes from their lives, past or present.

Whenever someone expressed unfinished business or something about a relationship that I sensed should be pursued further and more deeply, we would do a *role reversal.* Either that person would choose who would play their son, daughter-in-law, helper, friend, neighbor, grandchild, doctor etc., or I would ask one of the people on the staff to be that person. This is known in psychodrama as the *auxiliary ego* or we would simply have the person involved imagine the person he or she was in conflict with, to be seated on an *empty chair.*

The person in the group who was the focus of our enactment is called the *protagonist.*

We *concretized* with scarves, puppets, and objects in the room. *Concretizing* occurs when I ask the participant to translate abstract feelings into something tangible that we can see. In this way, they gain a deeper understanding of what is going on.

We did *sociometry* by raising our hands from 0 to 10 to show how much we identified with a statement.

There was a lot of *mirroring* throughout our sessions. This occurs when what is said or enacted is reflected back to the person from the director or someone else in our circle or when the person sees other people reenacting his scene for him.

Guided imagery is done by creating a relaxed atmosphere through making the participants feel very comfortable and then guiding them through the use of your voice, music or anything that will help create a mood and help the people focus on or *find* whatever specific image you would like to elicit.

An example of guided imagery was when the participants were asked to imagine photos from their lives, from imaginary picture albums which we would then bring to life.

We did *vignettes,* (short scenes) which were followed by *sharing.* This is a psychodramatic technique where we talk about ourselves and talk about how we have connected to what we have just witnessed. The protagonist listens to the sharing and is comforted and encouraged by hearing the stories of other members of our group. This technique helps the protagonist feel less exposed as the other members reveal their personal experiences.

We used *action* methods by *doing* in every possible way and not just talking.

People in the group and the young volunteers served as *auxiliary egos* – they are actually the actors in the enactment.

There were many incidents of connection that were so strong, the people in the circle experienced, what Moreno called, *tele* – a kind of two-way empathy.

The volunteers who took roles ended their roles by *de-roling* – announcing their names and stating they were no longer the role that they have just played.

Sometimes we fantasized situations, such as "The Forest". In psychodrama, this is called *surplus reality*. This is when we transcend reality and pretend.

There are a lot of similarities in Kohut's and Moreno's approach to therapy. This could explain my affinity to both of them and why many of the terms you will encounter come from the work of Heinz Kohut. Born in Vienna in 1913, Heinz Kohut was a psychoanalyst and a renowned self-psychologist, who had a huge impact on my work. He moved to the United States and died in Chicago in 1981. A major part of my work is based on how I understood and interpreted some of the concepts from Heinz Kohut's self-theory. These concepts are *empathy, twinship, mirroring and grandiosity*. They are basic to the therapeutic benefits of using drama with our population. These terms will also be explained in simple lay terms in the section in PART III: Understanding Heinz Kohut.

Following are examples of exercises using psychodramatic techniques and tools that were used in our 75-minute sessions. Some of these exercises are described briefly and some stand out as so beneficial that it is important to see the responses in detail. There are sample elaborations in this section and more to follow afterward. I am so thankful that, close to the beginning of our process, I realized that this documentation is precious and should be recorded. I bought a special, beautiful bound notebook and asked our volunteers to record what was being said.

This has turned out to be four large volumes over the past five years with the spelling, penmanship and grammar of at least twenty different people from ages ranging 18–70. Moreno said that psychodrama is the *Theater of Truth*, and this documentation certainly proves this (Image 3.1).

The Empty Chair

"Sitting in the empty chair is. . ."

- Someone to whom you want to say I'm sorry.
- Someone who needs to apologize to you.
- Someone with whom you have unfinished business.

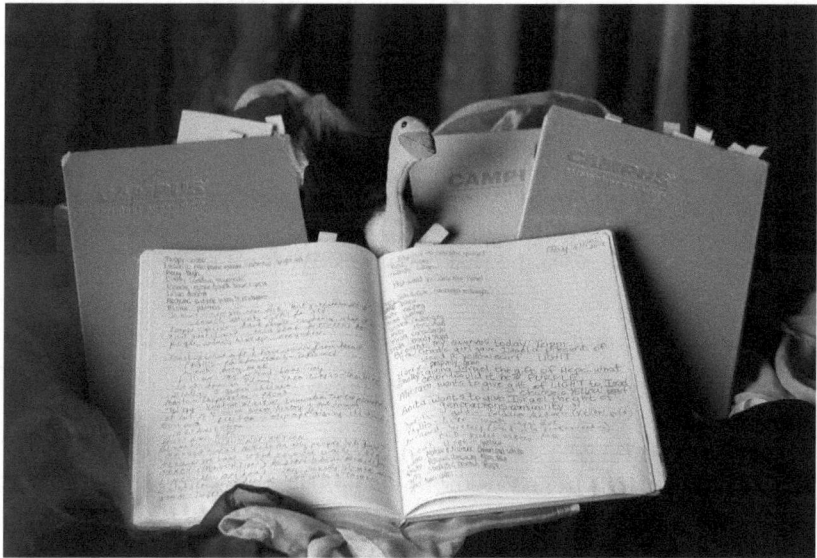

Image 3.1 Precious documentation

- Someone you want to thank, bless, complain to, compliment, or just meet again for a short visit.
- Any object that can tell us something about you.
- A part of your body with a complaint about you.

For example, sitting in the Empty Chair is a grandchild.

(This subject arose because I brought one of my granddaughters, Amalia, to the Center to volunteer for a day.) Through this *role reversal*, we could deepen our understanding about conflict between the generations.

This is how this session is built.

- The brightly colored scarves are laid out on the table at the head of our circle.
- Introduce today's subject, for example, "Grandparents".
- Tell the Group: "Find an adjective that describes what kind of a grandparent I am and complete the sentence 'I am a _____ grandparent . . .'" (see list of the adjectives below).
- Let's use these adjectives and more words that define what the word grandparent means to us. Select a scarf that "says" this for you, and then, with the scarves, let's sculpt our grandparent scarf sculpture. Now, by looking at this sculpture, we can *see* our association with this word.

As the participants choose a scarf that symbolizes the adjective they have found, and we see our ideal grandparent taking shape, they also gain new options to describe their individual grandparenting. (I had checked previously that they were all grandparents.)

This was a warm-up. Now the group is ready to *work*. Proceed to build the session with the following statement:

- If my grandchild were sitting in this *Empty Chair*, what would I say to him or her? What would he or she say to me? Find a typical sentence. Let's hear. Give us some real examples. We want to know."

Example and Elaboration: Grandparents

The participants give the following adjectives:

> generous, caring, happy, role-model, well-meaning, old fashioned, honest, truthful, too generous, not judgmental, critical, great, practicing-in-training, constructive, educational, absentee, sick, easy going, old, playful, entertaining, worried, a keeper of things – still has shoes that are thirty years old – story-telling, dedicated, loving, creative, doting, old fashioned.

Ask the group if anyone would like a chance to talk to a grandchild here and now – *psychodramatically*? They understand this sentence. they have heard it in numerous sessions, "In psychodrama, we can meet anyone we want!" This group has witnessed this many times. They are very familiar with this technique and know how to use it and benefit from it.

With a lot of role reversals, where he plays both Harvey, the man who stated that he was an old-fashioned grandfather, volunteers. My teenage granddaughter Amalia sits in the chair and as an *auxiliary ego*, plays the role of his teenage granddaughter. He opens up and complains to her that there is a need for more communication between them. My granddaughter does a terrific job. She knows what to say and exactly how to express it. She uses the information that Harvey offers. She affirms that he is old fashioned. It is time for him to update his mobile phone after ten years. She is giving it to him loud and clear! Her day at Melabev has turned out to be very significant in our relationship. (I am glad she has never told me off like that!)

With a lot of role reversals, where he plays both himself and his granddaughter and hears his text, Harvey understands and internalizes that he is, indeed, old fashioned. He needs a smartphone so that they can WhatsApp. His granddaughter promises to learn more spoken English, and he promises to try to learn Hebrew. All of this will create better communication. He understands that there is a strong desire for communication, love, interest, concern and caring on both sides.

In these role reversals, he recites all of his granddaughter's text when he plays her role. As in all psychodrama enactments, there is sharing afterward when the other members talk about how they connected to what they have just witnessed. This makes Harvey understand that he is not the only one in our Group with a communication issue with grandchildren. Most of their grandchildren speak too fast, too much Hebrew, swallow their words or are too busy texting with their smartphones! He is not alone!

Roles

There is one sentence that I heard at a psychodrama Zoom workshop on using psychodrama to treat trauma survivors given by Sylvia Israel[1] where she states that for Moreno, "Who we are is the sum of the roles we play." This is so basic and yet, we never really think about our roles in life.

> "Who we are is the sum of the roles we play."

According to Sylvia Israel, for Moreno, "health is to be able to play a lot of roles and to create new roles when necessary". All of our participants have to create new roles in their old age because of their increasingly serious cognition and health conditions. One of these roles is to be a participant in a psychodrama group at Melabev. This was most definitely new for them.

The Importance of Working on Roles for the Elderly

Role-playing, role reversals, represent a small part of working with our roles. The grandfather role in the above session shows how role-playing helped Harvey understand his need to make some changes in his behavior in the role of grandfather. Helping the people in this group examine their behavior and attitudes in a variety of roles gives them important information about themselves and helps them understand intricacies in their relationships with all the other people in their lives, and above all, it helps them cope and adjust to their challenging situations.

---

1 Sylvia Israel, LMFT, RDT/BCT, is cofounder of Bay Area Moreno Institute, IMAGINE! The Center for Creativity & Healing and Bay Area Playback Theatre. She teaches graduate students at the California Institute of Integral Studies (CIIS) and Kansas State University, and maintains a private practice in San Francisco, California

So much has been written about Role Theory in psychodrama and drama therapy. In his seminal work, *Drama Therapy: Concepts, Theories and Practices* (1994, p. 46) Robert Landy, a leading drama therapist, states that "a general, more philosophical purpose of drama therapy is to increase the client's repertory of roles and his ability to play a single role more fully".

Tian Dayton, a leading psychodramatist, states that "psychological health is associated with the ability to move in and out of a variety of roles with relative fluidity". Dayton, *The Drama Within: Psychodrama and Experiential Therapy* (p. 21). It is important to stress that since this book is a guide, I will be focusing only on what directly impacts our population.

The following techniques can be used after the session where we sculpt a grandparent and then use the *empty chair* to develop this subject. I say:

"Let's make a list of the real roles we have in our lives."

The participants are very impressed with the number and variety of roles they have listed; they are rich in roles. Just to give you an idea of the range of roles I will list a few:

Parent, spouse, grandparent, great grandparent, sister, brother, patient, boss of an aide, cousin, aunt, friend, neighbor, member of Melabev, consumer, customer, adviser, fixer, knitter, traveler, bereaved parent, widow, widower, mender, citizen, member of a community, voter, cantor, Rabbi, teacher, writer, reader, step-mother, step-father, etc.

For homework, I ask them to think of other roles that we might have forgotten. They immediately add a few; divorcee, a member of a WhatsApp group and many more;. the excitement of this discovery is tangibly in the air. Yes, we are rich in roles.

I look at our list, and show how impressed I am and I suggest that we find a way to examine our attitudes, behavior and conflicts in some of these roles.

- What kind of parent, grandparent, sibling, friend, neighbor, patient, cousin, and so on, am I?
- We work on the role of friend. It is relatively safe and non-risky. I say, "Give yourself an adjective in this role."

I am a ____friend.

Some examples of their adjectives: helpful, listening, talkative, complaining, confiding, telephone talking, trusting, distant, loyal, etc.

- I place two chairs in the center of our circle. I elaborate and demonstrate. The chair on my right is (subjectively) positive. The one on my left is (subjectively) negative. In the *positive* chair I am proud of the way I behave in one of these roles. In the *negative* chair I am not happy, proud or satisfied with the way I behave in this role. I say: "Let's hear what you have to say in each chair."

I demonstrate with the role of a friend. I jump from chair to chair as I rattle off why I am a good friend and why I am a terrible friend. Once the participants see me do this, they are ready to give it a try and we move on to other roles.

Examining Our Roles

- What are some roles you would like to add to your list?
- What is your favorite role?
- Are there any roles you would like to remove?
- What roles are easy for you?
- What roles are difficult for you?
- Can you invest more effort in any of these roles?
- Do you invest too much energy in any of these roles?
- In what roles are you not alone?

Many of these ideas were inspired by Tian Dayton's book, *The Drama Within* (1994).

I must add that all through my career, whenever I did this exercise with a group or at a workshop that I conducted, I discovered my own needs and understood my own conflicts so much better. Additional roles that I wanted to add to my list, over the years, were:

> To lead a psychodrama group. That was many years and many groups ago.
> To be a grandmother. That was twenty-five years ago and twenty-four grandchildren ago.
> To be an author. Well, you all know when that wish came true.

Projection Via Puppets: Elaboration

All my life, puppets were for puppet shows – my puppet shows. I even performed and toured with an educational puppet theatre. Puppets were my voice through ventriloquism.

I always had two puppets and they expressed two sides of my personality so well that it surprised me. They were my therapy from age 12; they were my *Theater of Truth.*

I did not know this until I studied psychodrama and learned about projection.

Why puppets? Often it is easier to get to our truth via projection. A puppet can express feelings that we would never admit to. There is a safe aesthetic distance from ourselves.

This is true, especially with adults. But would it be true for our group?? I had to try it out!

I bring in an assortment of animal puppets (Images 3.2–3.4).

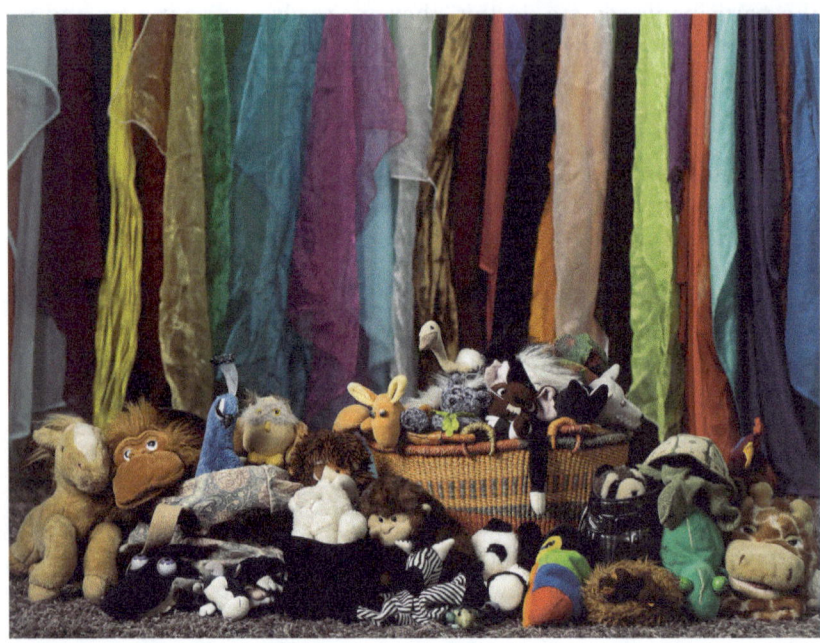

Image 3.2 Puppets are safe and unthreatening – puppets tell the truth

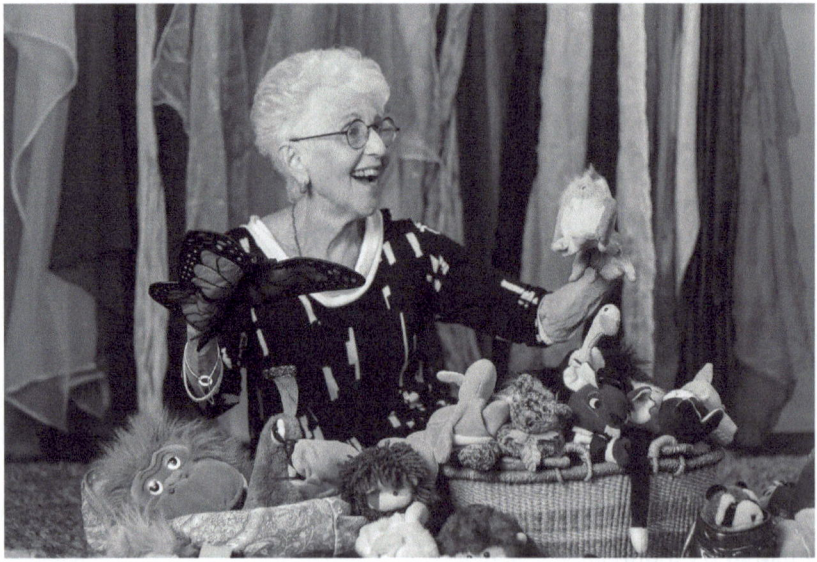

Image 3.3 . . . and are so much fun

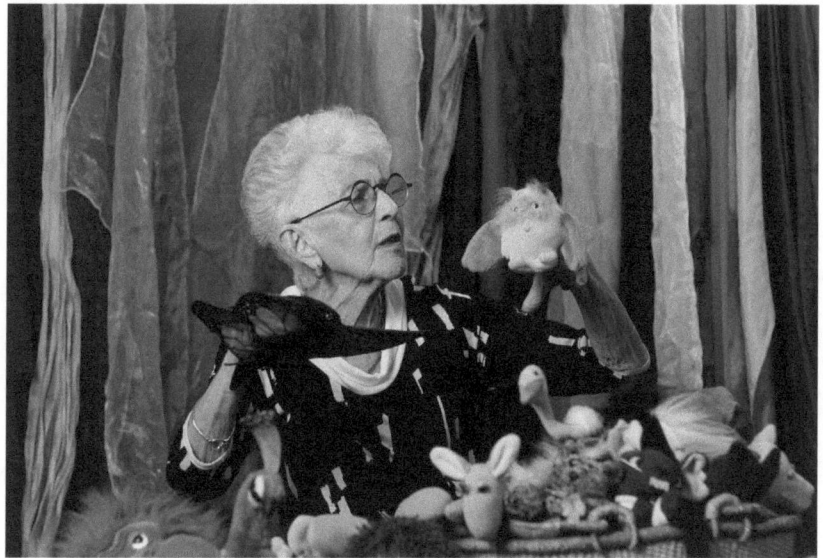

Image 3.4 . . . and so easy to talk to

They are set up on a table in the center of the circle. Everyone is seated around the table. This is a new setting for our session as usually we are seated in a large circle without a table. I introduce some of the puppets so that our group can see the variety. I even let some of the puppets talk for the fun of it. We are ready to begin our session.

I say to everyone, "Pick a puppet that depicts how the world sees you." These are some of their choices:

- Peacock = colorful
- Turtle = always sleeping
- Butterfly = what is left for me to do? Flutters above everything. Sees all, but is not involved.
- Dog = loyal
- Turkey = people see me as a clown.
- Ostrich = head in the ground.
- Zebra = I have my own characteristics.

I can see that our group members are investing a lot of thought in their selections. They really want to know how the world sees them. They identify with the puppets that are selected. Surprisingly, this is not difficult for them.

Simmy, the 91-year-old male psychology professor, selects a raccoon hidden inside a garbage can (Image 3.5).

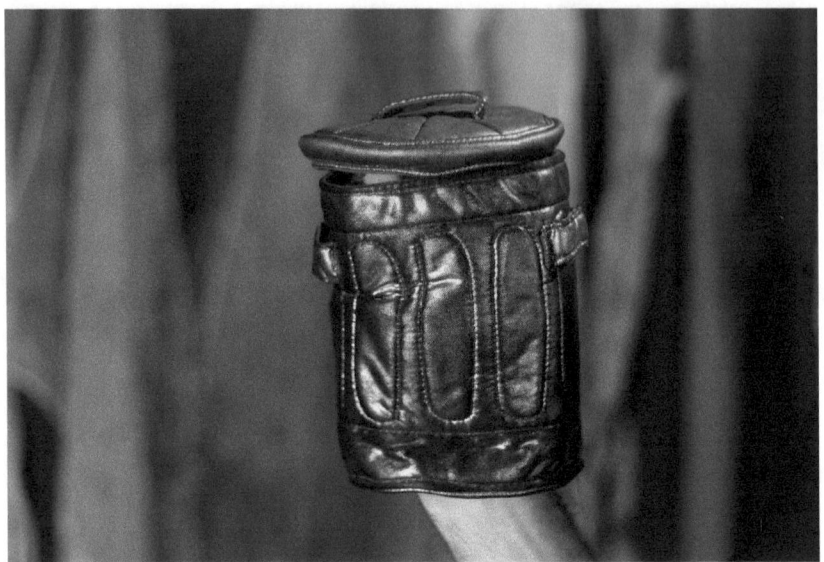

Image 3.5

The puppet starts talking. Its movements are delicate. They express such timidity and sadness. "No one sees me. I left. It is as if I don't exist anymore. I feel invisible" (Images 3.6 and 3.7).

This begs to be developed into what becomes a very moving psychodrama. I ask Simmy, "Who *does* see you?" And he answers, "My wife, Joanne." He picks Avi, a member of our Group, to play his wife. He role-reverses with Avi. Then, he plays his wife, Joanne, and Avi becomes him, Simmy. What develops is amazing. I ask *her* (Simmy) "Did he disappear?" And *she* answers, "He can walk. He can talk. He can flirt with girls. He tries to read."

I ask her to tell *him* that. Simmy (as Joanne) turns to Avi – who is still in the role of Simmy and continues with the following unforgettable text.

> All the people like you. They admire you. They remember that you opened the Department of Psychology at the university. So many of your former students and colleagues come to visit you. They all read your books and articles and want to discuss things with you. No way did you disappear! You are very present and visible in their lives (Image 3.8).

Simmy says this empowered statement psychodramatically and when he role reverses and hears Avi repeat this text, as his wife Joanne, he replies very emotionally, with the biggest smile, "You must be right."

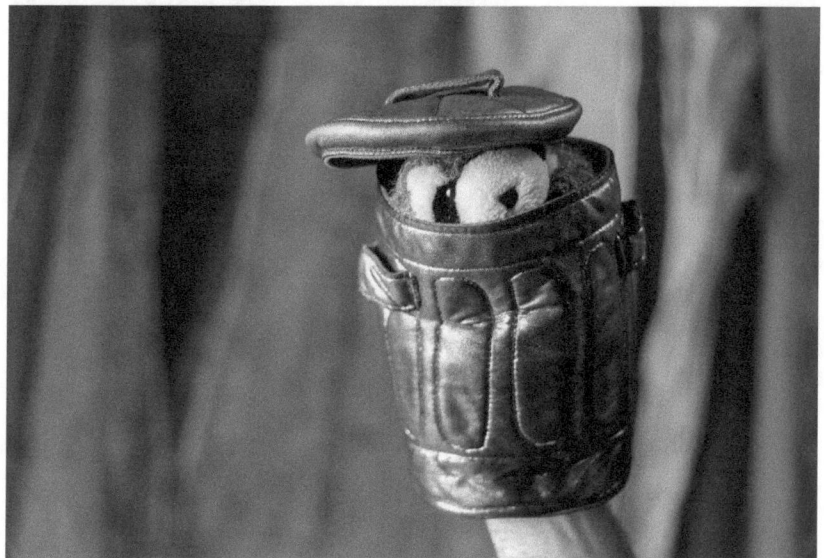

Image 3.6

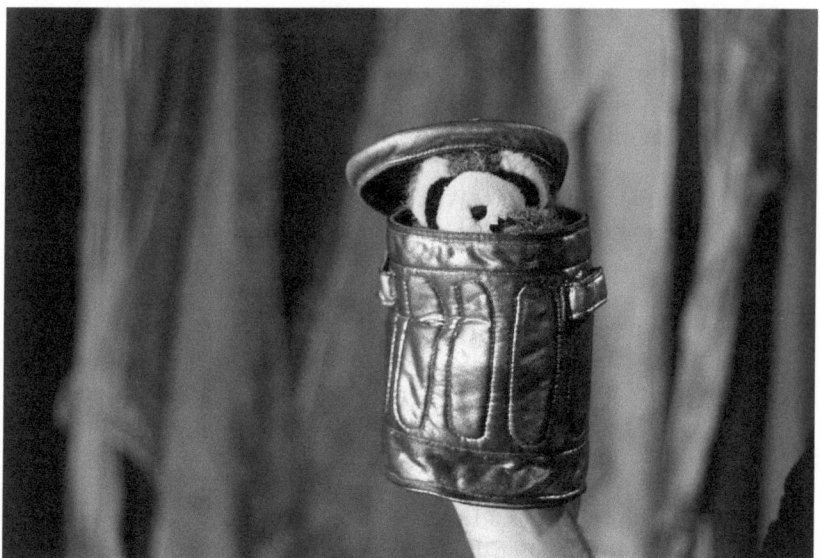

Image 3.7 "No-one sees me"

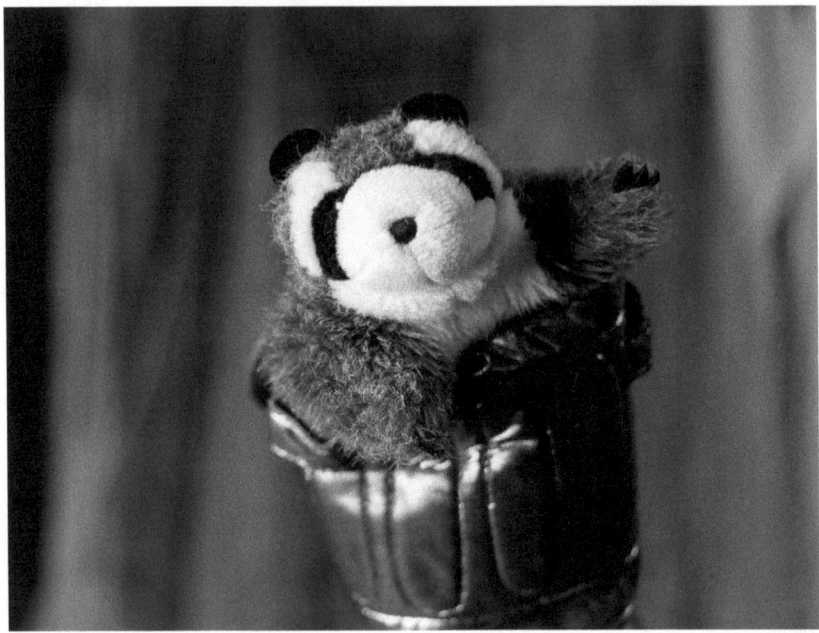

Image 3.8 "Looks like I did not disappear"

In comparison with how he is described when you meet our members, as "always smiling and he didn't know why". This time, his smile is one of recognition, awareness and pride. And he knows why he is smiling.

After this, I then ask them, "What puppets have traits that you need?" Following are some examples of what these beautiful animal puppets are projecting for the participants:

- Turtle = "I have to slow down."
- Monkey = "I have to learn to be more playful."
- Puppy = "I want people to see the soft tender side of me."
- Peacock = "I have to be less shy. I have to open up my feathers and show the world – me."
- Jaguar = "I need a Jaguar to feel strong."
- Rabbit in the Hat = "I had a friend who survived Auschwitz by doing magic tricks for the guards. This exercise made me think about him because I need to pull the rabbit out of the hat too, to show my unique traits."
- Dalmatian = "I need a loyal friend to be around me all the time."
- Fish = "I need to go with the flow."

I then ask, "What puppet shows who I *really* am?" Here are some of their replies.

- Elephant = thick skinned.
- Butterfly = fluttering.
- Chameleon = changing according to the situation.
- Dog = loyal
- Owl = wise and old.
- Bumble Bee = I can sting.
- Rabbit in the Hat = very creative.
- Turtle = I need protection.
- Little lamb = very vulnerable.

In the future, I would like to bring these beautiful puppets back into the room. These puppets became the "Theater of Truth" for our participants.

Sharing – From My Process With Adolescents

As I have stated, many of these exercises are variations of exercises I have been using with younger populations. One example that I would like to share here occurred with a group of eighth-grade girls with life-changing results. These girls were selected, by the school adviser, to participate in a psychodrama therapy group with me once a week. They all had emotional problems that affected their social interactions and their ability to learn. They needed to develop self-confidence and social skills. The goal of this group was to enhance their self-image and help them to blossom along with their potential.

The puppets were used as described above but I added another exercise that was a game changer for one girl in this group. She was tall, beautiful, impressive, and apparently very bright. Surprisingly, she was quiet and introverted. She hardly spoke. Communicating with her through words was definitely challenging. Her breakthrough came with a simple exercise with masks (Image 3.9).

Each girl in the group picked a mask, gave it an entire identity, wore it and became the character it depicted. She picked a mask of an elegant woman. I asked her to enter the room as this woman. All of a sudden, her height enabled her to become a truly majestic woman, and her posture, stature and body language were transformed by the mask. When I interviewed the character she had created, guess what? She spoke. We could see her elegance and we could also hear a grand courtly voice that spoke with authority and confidence, via the mask. As soon as she removed the mask, she shriveled up and stopped speaking. At our next session, I brought in these same puppets and did all of the above-listed exercises. I added another exercise by requesting that they pick a puppet of their choice. Any puppet to which they felt a deep connection. She picked a small delicate lamb (Image 3.10).

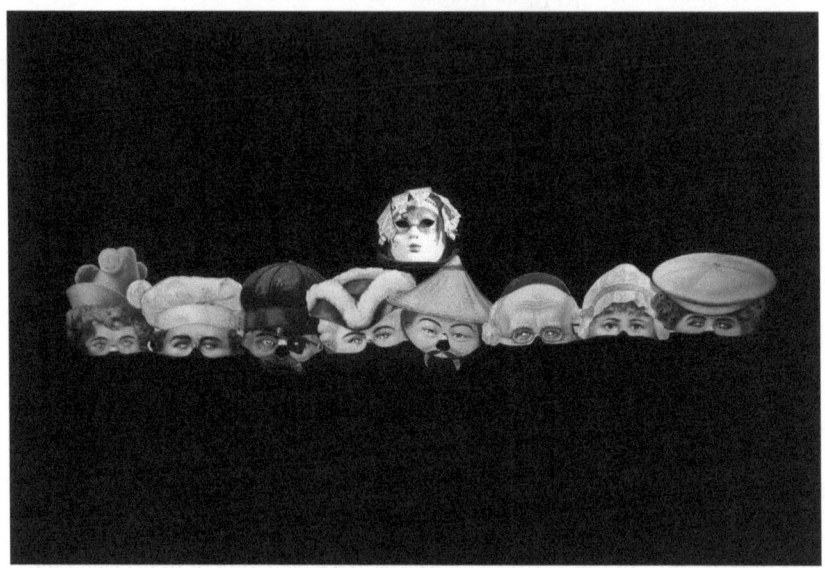

Image 3.9 The transformative magic of masks

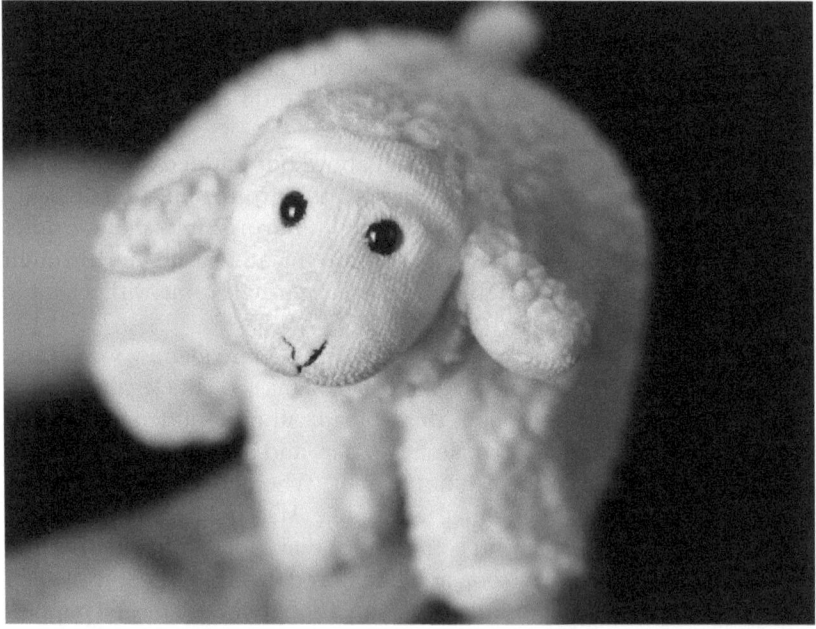

Image 3.10 Delicate lamb

The girls became a therapy group of animal puppets. We had a lion, giraffe, zebra, a colorful parrot, an owl, elephant, a Dalmatian, monkey, a scary crocodile and our timid little lamb. I told the girls that for the next half hour we would be a support group of these puppets. I asked everyone to think of a problem their puppet might have. I then asked the puppets to share their problem with the rest of our puppet group. We had a scary crocodile who had no friends because everyone was afraid of her. The lion shared a similar problem, and they decided to become friends. The girl, described above, was playing the lamb. She was warmed up. Something happened and suddenly we heard the lamb's voice expressing a deep need. The lamb said, "No-one sees me" (like Simmy, mentioned above). The zebra replied, "I will give you my stripes, then everyone will definitely see you. I am certain of that." The little lamb said, "Thank you but stripes won't help me." So, the colorful parrot offered its bright colors. "With all of my colors, you will definitely be seen." Then the little lamb made a statement that I will never forget. She expressed herself very clearly, authentically and emotionally. "You don't understand", she said, "I don't need help to be seen from the outside, it's my inside that no-one sees!"

The session continued and everyone was treated to a lot of information on the *inside* of this little lamb, who was no longer timid and had a lot to say about herself and her experience of *not being seen*. Our psychodrama group became a circle of trust for her and slowly, she also opened up outside of the group sessions. This book is not about teenagers but this story demonstrates the transformative power of puppets and the intrinsic magic of the use of masks in a drama session.

The Benefits of Anonymity: The Hat of Fear

Explanation of the Technique

I bring in a very impressive hat and announce, "This hat is called *The Hat of Fear*."[2] This statement arouses their curiosity, and I then ask: "Why? Because as soon as I put this hat on my head, I feel strong and confident, without fear."

I demonstrate by strutting to the center of our circle feeling very self-assured and I declare, "You see? It *absorbs* our fear (Images 3.11–3.13).

> I am going to place it in the center of our circle. I am going to give each of you a piece of paper on which you will write, anonymously, without signing your name, your response to whatever I ask you. This

---

2 This tool was taken from P. Wilkins, Sage Publications, London, 1999, (p. 55). Wilkins' terminology is "Fear in the Hat". My recollection of this exercise was "Hat of Fear" and that works for me.

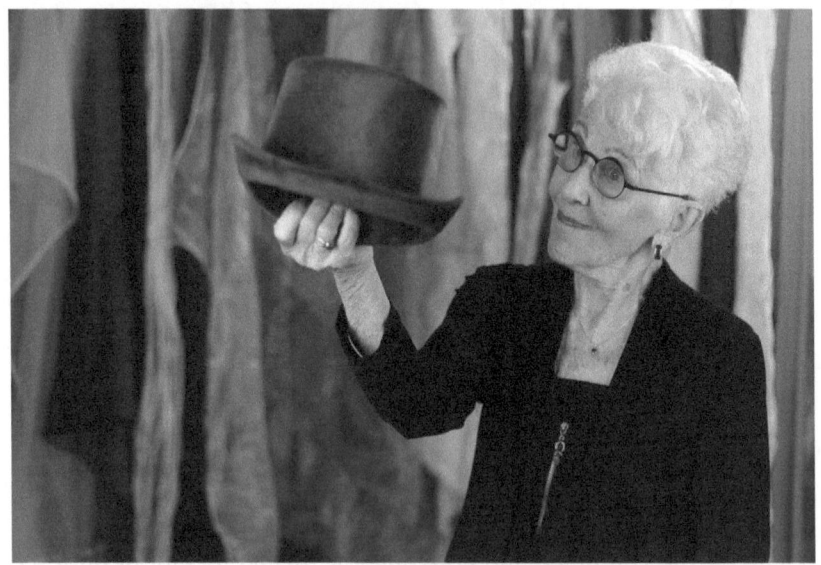

Image 3.11

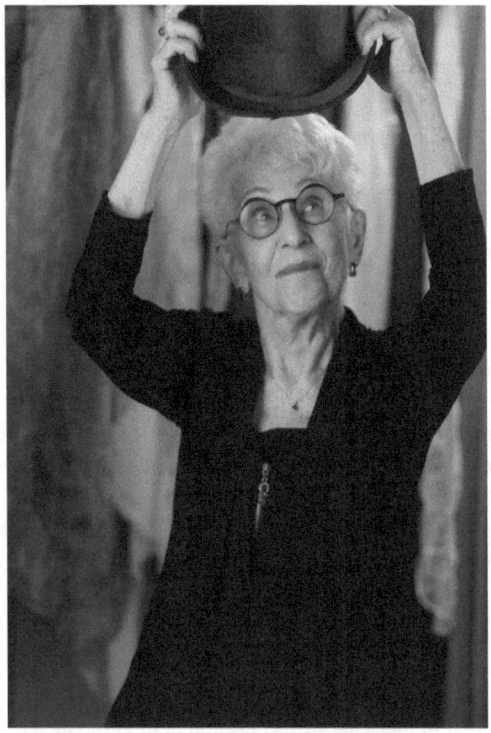

Image 3.12 The *Hat of Fear* – encourages authentic, unabashed self-expression

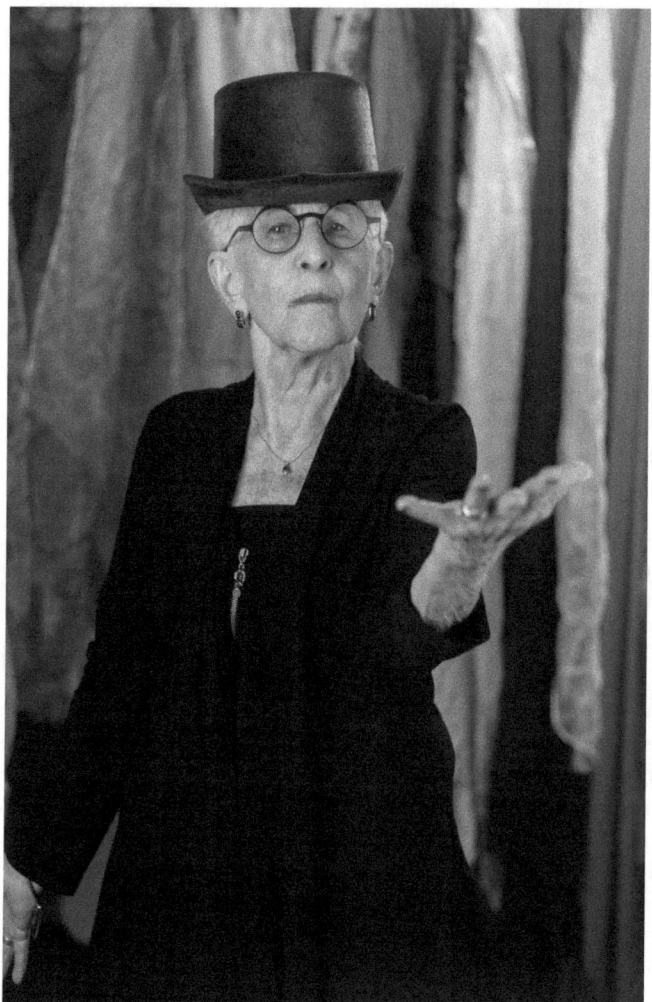

Image 3.13 It absorbs all my fears

is the secret to the success of this technique; the anonymity enables total freedom of expression. I continue, "No-one in the group will know who wrote what we will be hearing. Our volunteers will help anyone who needs assistance writing.

For example: Write something that makes you feel uneasy in this group. All the notes will be folded and put into The Hat of Fear and then each of you will pick a note from the hat. You will then read aloud whatever is written on your paper. This is a form of *role reversal* because you will read the note as if *you* wrote it. We will hear every-one's answer, and it will become a group language.

This is an example of *mirroring* that is audio because everyone in the group will HEAR what they wrote and only the person who wrote that note will recognize his words. This exercise works beautifully with every age group. I have used it to give expression to many deep, uncomfortable, embarrassing, confusing and conflicting issues in groups.

Suggestions for exercises utilizing *The Hat of Fear*:

- What would I like to work on in a psychodrama enactment or vignette?
- A compliment I would like to hear.
- A compliment that I can give to myself. No modesty allowed. (You cannot compliment others, if you don't know your own strengths)
- What would I like to change in myself?
- What activities in this center need improvement?

I am elaborating on a session using this technique in order to show the amount of sincere unabashed expression when there is anonymity.

Example of a Session: What Do I Have to Do to Be the Best Me Possible?

It is the start of a new year and I bring in my peacock puppet (Image 3.14) and my "Hat of Fear" (Image 3.15).

As concrete inspiration, I show the group how the peacock puppet spreads its feathers and shows its magnificence (Images 3.16 and 3.17).

I tell them, "Now the peacock is the best it can be. I would like you to think about what you have to do to show your feathers, to realize your potential, to be the best you can be." I reframe and say, "Think about what do I have to do to make the New Year greeting, *A Happy Healthy Fulfilling New Year*, happen for me?"

Everyone gets a piece of paper and writes their answer. The staff is available to anyone who needs help. The responses are written without their names so that each slip of paper is anonymous. The folded papers are put into my *Hat of Fear* (Image 3.18).

I mix them up and pass the hat around. Everyone picks a slip of paper, reads it to themselves, (some with assistance from the staff) and then we *hear* what was written. As each person reads out what is written on the note he or she picked out of the hat, each participant hears what they personally wrote. In this way, we can learn from all the responses and even gain new options. Moreover, everyone in the group experiences *audio mirroring*.

Following is what is written anonymously. You will notice that many of the participants reveal more than one goal.

What do I have to do to be the best me possible?

- Show my inner beauty and improve my life in the coming year.
- Be myself proudly.

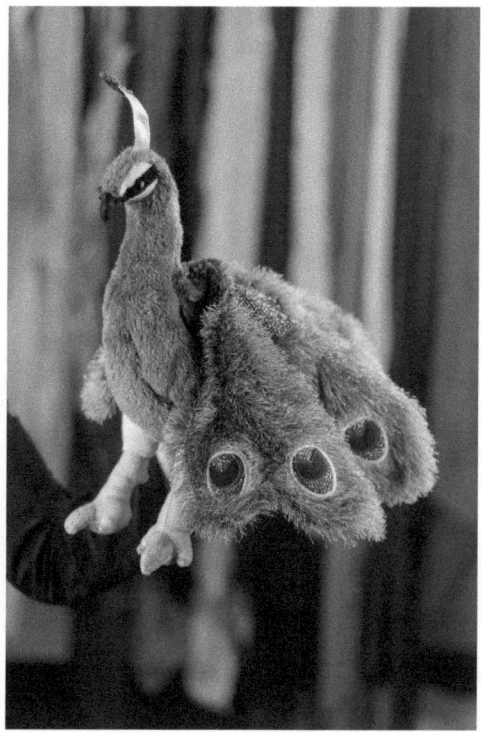

Image 3.14 Peacock puppet

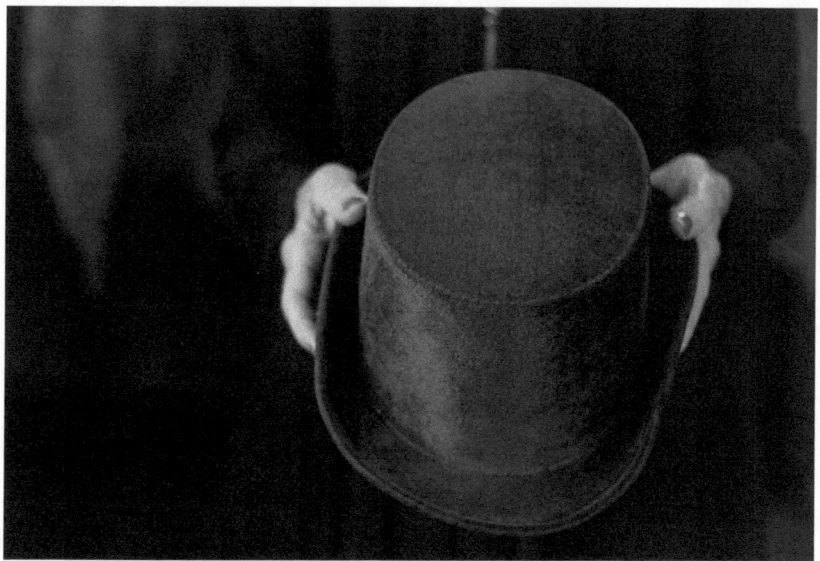

Image 3.15 My "*Hat of Fear*"

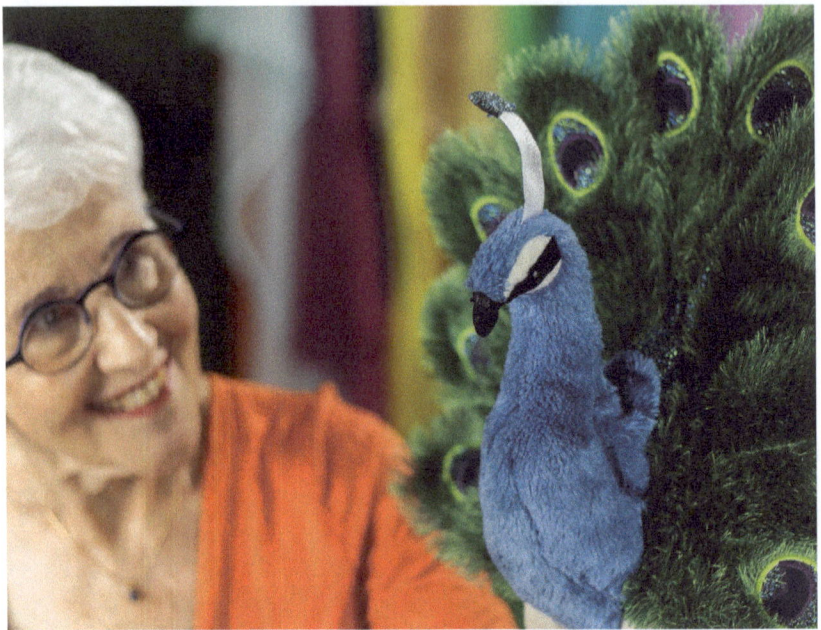

Image 3.16 The peacock displays its plume

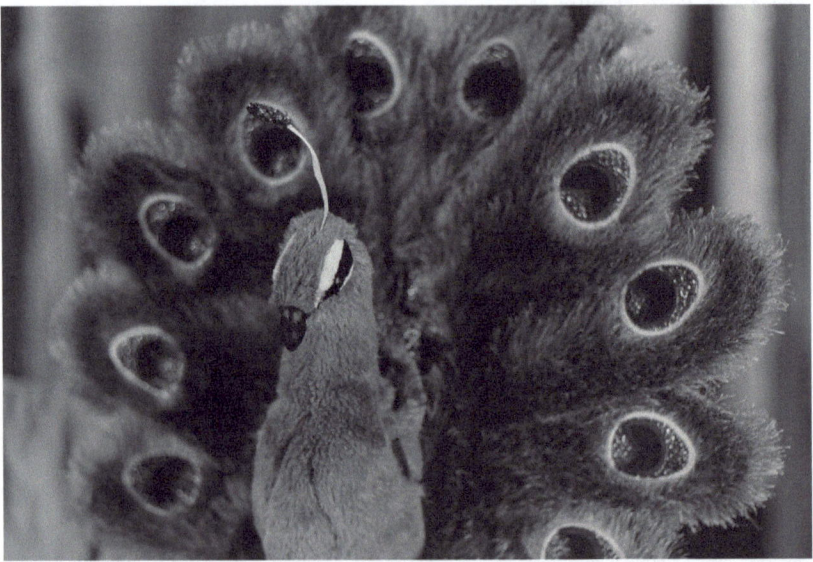

Image 3.17 The peacock shows its magnificence

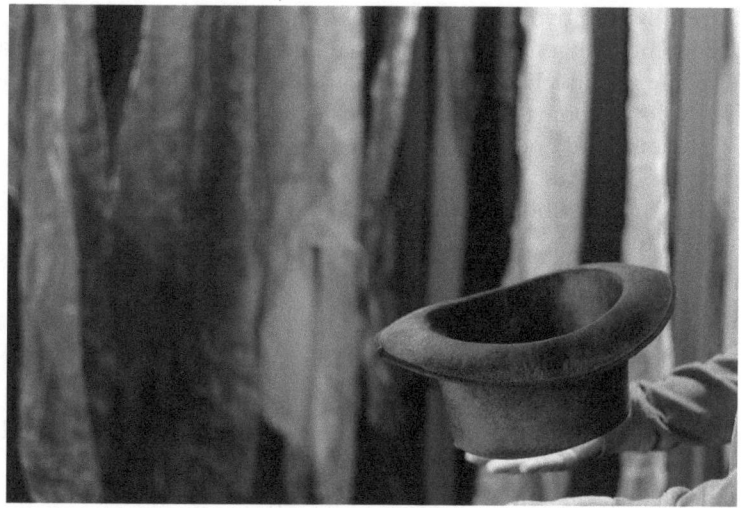

Image 3.18 Hat of Fear ready for anonymous notes

- Judge people more favorably.
- Show people love and compassion.
- Not allow my fears to control me or stop me from living my life to the fullest.
- Be really interested in *me*. To hear *me*, to see *me*.
- Keep appreciating all that I am and all that I am blessed with and let that be enough for now. If more blessings come, I won't complain.
- Give more charity.
- Invite more people to my home.
- Invite Sabbath guests and holiday guests.
- I need to accept my age and limitations.
- I need to not compare.
- I need to not lose my self-confidence so easily and remember who I am.
- Relief from the excruciating pain I've had for the past few years.
- I have to stop complaining.
- I have to overcome the sadness of the loss of the people in the past and try even harder to enjoy the people in my life today.
- I have to accept the fact that I have to lean on others.
- I have to straighten out things that I made a mess of.
- I need to be the best me possible.
- Take another language course in Hebrew so that I can communicate with my grandchildren.
- Order and try out a new hearing aid.
- This coming year, I want to be on the giving side, not on the receiving side. And only in good health.

- At this stage in my life, I need to be the best grandfather possible; carefully attentive to my grandchildren.
- I want my youngest daughter to get a spouse and become pregnant and give me a grandchild like the peacock that opens up and encourages seduction. I come to Melabev not to achieve and I do enjoy myself.
- To be nice and good.
- Try to be a better *mensch* than I was the day before. Hillel said it all. "Love thy neighbor like thyself."
- To be honest.
- To be sincere.
- To be truthful.
- To be considerate.
- To be clean at home.
- Be aware, conscious of what I am doing.
- I would like to think what the other person needs and feels and be there for them.
- I hope in the coming year to be less judgmental towards others.
- I hope to try to exercise more and not be lazy about it.
- To try and keep in touch with friends and family that I feel I have neglected recently.
- I want to love unconditionally.
- I want to emulate the action of two role models. They keep their word and I try to emulate their actions.
- Don't sweat the small stuff. I have a hard time telling the differences between what is small and what is big.
- Spend a lot more time exercising, walking and pushing myself to do things that are hard for me.
- I need more patience with my husband and with people around me. I keep trying and hope I will be able to improve in the coming year.
- I hope to encourage my children in many different ways.
- Try not to bother my children for anything or be a burden to them. I want to remain independent.

The following week I read all these brave honest responses out loud and ask all of the participants to raise their hands in a show of 0–10 for each statement to see how many identify with what was anonymously written. This sociometric exercise develops a profound sense of belonging as our group members look around the circle and see where all the hands are.

Then with each response, we discuss:

- Who can help us accomplish this goal?
- Who is making it problematic?
- Who should we meet in the *empty chair* in order to address this insight?
- We also worked on whether we are a burden to our children when we ask for help.

Think of the array of options the participants have just received from this exercise at the beginning of the New Year. They are making choices. They gain a sense of freedom from their disabilities.

Hat of Fear allows us to talk about the issues that are difficult to talk about. These anonymous notes, in the hat, are the gateway to our Theater of Truth.

Psychodrama à Deux

After working for at least a year, I feel that my group is ready to do some work in pairs. This is a major leap forward. Some of them need assistance but most of them enjoy the intimacy of two.

I have always been uncomfortable when I participate in a workshop and we are instructed to pick a partner. As a result, I always avoid this situation, even with children, or maybe, especially with children. I simply arrange the members so that they are paired with someone else each time. They could sit according to the first letter of their first name or according to the date of birth. They could be paired with someone who is wearing the same color as they are. Any criterion works, as long as the outcome is dynamic, and it usually is. I give them a reason to be together as a couple in the exercise.

Working in pairs induces a sense of deep comfort, belonging and identification. Kohut calls this closeness *twinship*. Many group leaders make the mistake of asking every pair to simply talk to each other about anything. This can be very awkward. The conversations will sound something like "uh, heh, urr, um, etc.". Or we will have complete silence and awkward laughter – not to mention, a sudden rush to the bathroom. If the pairs are given a specific subject to explore together, the conversation will flow immediately. They need a trigger to get started. This is true for all populations. It has nothing to do with cognition.

Exercises for Pairs

Here are some suggestions for topics to use in pairs that this group felt comfortable with and were able to initiate conversations:

• Tell your partner something nice or new that happened to you in the past week, month, year or since the last national or religious holiday, or any significant date. Now your partner will tell the group your story and you will listen. Then you will tell the group your partner's story. This is an example of audio *mirroring* where each person can hear what they have just said. Moreover, everyone gets to talk in front of the group more easily because they are not talking about themselves. They have the incentive to work very hard not to forget what their partner told them. Such a simple way to stimulate their memory, and so basic and essential for this group!

Suggestion: Often, when someone tells a story, ask them: If this story would be made into a book or a film what would its name or title be? The partner is also asked to think of an appropriate title. This can be followed up by opening the request to the entire group. If I have an inspiring title or name, I offer my suggestion. My hope is that they will focus on a central theme. This will help them consolidate all the facts and many of the details and remember the experience. Moreover, the storyteller receives a lot of significant *mirroring* (reflecting back) from the group.

- Tell your partner three traits that you have: one that you are proud of, one that you want to change or improve, one that helps you cope. Try to remember these three traits. If it is too difficult to remember, the staff will help you write it all down. Your partner will then introduce you to the group using these three traits.

As mentioned above, this can be examined sociometrically by raising of hands from 0 to 10: What traits were mentioned that you could have used to describe yourself but you didn't think of?

What traits were mentioned that you need?

- Now, let's do the same exercise again by switching roles. You tell us about your partner.
- Give your partner a compliment. Your partner will give you a compliment.

Drama Gift Shop

I describe the *Drama Gift Shop*, a popular drama therapy exercise. I tell the group that in the drama gift shop we can buy anything we want. If they are willing, we can even use the scarves to symbolize our purchase, because thankfully they are no longer considered "schmattes"! I emphasize that the time department in the Drama Gift Shop is extremely popular. For example: We can buy a watch that adds time to our day when we need it or are simply enjoying ourselves. There are clocks that wait till we are finished or ready. We can even rush or skip time, if necessary. We have a watch for every need, not to mention our array of clocks. These examples help our participants understand the options. The most moving gift ever bought in the *Drama Gift Shop* was bought by a 9-year-old boy. It was a heart made of plastic so that it would not break. Another young boy who was a twin with three more siblings at home bought a gift for his mother – a watch with many more hours on it so that his mom would have some time – for him!

Here's how it works:

A. is the buyer and B. is the sales-person. I tell the buyer to purchase a gift in the *Drama Gift Shop* for someone they love or care about deeply. Then I have them switch: B. is the buyer and A. is the salesperson.

I do this exercise in the holiday season when everyone's mind is on gifts. This is an opportunity to express the joy of giving and to recognize people who you appreciate.

Now, I tell the Group:

> Go to the *Drama Gift Shop* and buy something for yourself. Tell the salesperson enough about yourself so that he or she will know what to find for you in our amazing shop. Think of something that will help you. Take advantage of this incredible opportunity. We all love bargains and great finds when we shop. Go for it.

I still have to ease them into this new idea. So, as a trigger, I give some personal examples:

> "I bought shoes that look fashionable but feel and support like orthopedic shoes."
> "I bought a filter. It helps me say whatever comes to my mouth but filters out all the extraneous things that the person I am talking to does not need to hear." (I wish I could remember to use it!)

These examples are more than triggers. They encourage genuine authentic self-reflection. The participants come up with honest and helpful items. Just knowing that you need something is already helpful. Somebody buys a computer that can work by itself. One of the men blurts out: "I bought a machine that puts on socks for me!" Another person bought a tiny machine that fits in her pocket and helps her remember!

Working in Small Groups

Finding what we have in common and what makes us special.

* Find three to five things that you have in common with your partner. Find three to five things that you and your partner do *not* have in common. For this group two or three can be enough.
* Combine every two pairs into groups of four.
* All four have to find one thing they have in common and find a way to SHOW the rest of the group what that is. The rest of the group will join them if it also applies to them.

For example: All of us wear hearing aids. All of us have a caretaker. All of us have great-grandchildren. I then ask, "Who else wears a hearing aid, has a caretaker or has great grandchildren?" This criterion creates deeper bonding and more social cohesion.

* Each person in each group of four will then have to find one thing that is unique to him or her in their small group.

"Only I was a soldier."
"Only I love pets."
"Only I love to garden."
"Only I am allergic to gluten."
"Only I can play the piano."

- Return to the large circle and announce to the entire group your "Only I" statement. Maybe someone else from another group will say "me too". Now I ask the group to look around the room and try to think of something that they are certain will be unique to them:

"Only I had 3 wives."
"Only I lived in Hawaii."
"Only I was orphaned at birth and was raised by my grandmother."

So much personal information is shared here and it is so easy to reveal it to others.

Group Greeting Cards

It is the holiday season and we want to send a greeting card to someone or to a group: Our group is divided into sub-groups of three to four people. A volunteer works with each group.

- To whom do you collectively decide to send your greeting card?

Some of their examples: People in the hospital, children starting first grade, all the children in the country, someone in the government, all the new immigrants to Israel, the soldiers, the unemployed, newly-weds, new parents.

- What do you want to say to these people?
- Present your card to the entire group. It can be either written or dramatically acted out.

This is group work that develops cooperation, creativity, more intricate interaction, group sharing and group pride, which all blend into social cohesion. As an intimate group of 4, they are excited to present their product together to the entire Group.

Emotion Exercises

One thing we all have in common is a basic need to deal with our emotions and feelings however different they may be.

When I broach the subject of emotions, I bring in a package of homemade cards on which I have written the names of over fifty emotions and feelings. Before displaying them, I ask the group to simply announce emotions and feelings that they experience in their daily lives. We write them on our blackboard. We then expand our list by adding the emotions of other people in our lives. I remind them to think of all the people we have invited to sit in *the Empty Chair*. We further expand by thinking of people we pass in our daily lives; the cab drivers, clerks, sales people, technicians, nurses, passengers on a bus, and so forth . . . We then add emotions from the news, movies or books we have read. I then reveal all of my cards and we check if they have added to my homemade collection of emotion cards. Yes, they are rich in emotions.

Here is the list of emotions and feelings that we collected from the experiences and the inner world of our participants – some of which are unique to them. I decided to keep it the way they said it, in their sincere, authentic vernacular:

Afraid, aggravated, alarmed, angry, annoyed, anxious astonished, betrayed, bitter, boastful, bored, cowardly, curious, cruel, cranky, crushed, delighted, depressed desire, despair, devastated, disappointed, discouraged, disgusted, ecstatic, embarrassed, empathic, empty!, enchanted, enthusiastic, envious, euphoric, excited, expectation, faith, fascinated, flabbergasted, frustrated, fulfilled, furious, grateful, greedy, guilty, happy, hate, horrified, hostile, humiliated, infatuation, innocence, intimidated, joy, jealous, lazy, left-out, liberated, lively, lonely, loyal, mean, obsessed, optimistic, outraged, overwhelmed, pacified, passionate, peaceful, pessimistic, pity, playful, pleased, proud, provoked, rage, regret, relief, resentment, sad, selfish, shame, shy, stupid, submissive, superior, surprised, sweet, temperamental, terrified, threatened, thrilled, tormented, tranquil, troubled, trust, uneasy, unhappy, unsure, useless, vengeful, vicious, warm, worthless, yearning.

We are now ready to examine this subject by showing and sharing. Begin by saying an emotion that comes to your head-and mouth and add a movement to accompany that emotion. The entire group mirrors that word and motion. The person to your right repeats what you said and did and adds another emotion and movement. The entire group mirrors both. Continue around the circle with each person repeating only the one person before them, and in the end, we have a chorus and dance of twenty emotions said and enacted.

For example: I say "anger" and poke my fist into my other hand in addition to making a grimace with my face. The entire group mirrors anger.

The person to my right repeats my word and movement and adds "love" and makes a hugging movement with her arms. The entire group repeats both anger and love. There is a sense of accomplishment and creative group satisfaction and pride.

When I was asked to work with this group, the member of staff responsible for them, Jennie, their leader, had this as her goal: An activity that will help these people talk about their feelings. She instinctively knew that this could best be accomplished through some form of drama. She was so right. This group loved all the emotion exercises. It was a direct vehicle for touching something that was buried deep inside them in a lonely place and yearning to be released and shared. This release is essential if an emotion is locked inside of us. I will never forget the little boy who was in a children's group I was leading way back in 1975. When I asked the youngsters to share when they are angry, he said, "I am never angry! Everyone is always angry at me!" I am certain that helping him touch his anger and frustration and identify with the responses of the other members of this young group was a game changer for him.

- Give a participant a card with an emotion written on it. (We have over fifty emotion cards! They are surprised by the quantity.) That person will then tell a personal story with that emotion, or act out that emotion, or make up a story with that emotion in it. The group will guess what emotion is being expressed and will then share their connection to that emotion.
- Scatter a bunch of cards with different emotions written on them on the floor. Ask for a volunteer to tell us a story and the rest of the group can then tell the story teller what emotion(s) they think were expressed in that story.
- This exercise becomes more creative and original and actually more therapeutic when you tell the group that today we are going to pretend we are all birds. Instruct them to look at the cards on the floor and, as a bird, tell a story involving one of the emotions. I could write a book of short stories from all the stories told by the birds I have met over the years in all of my groups.
- One person leaves the room and the group picks an emotion. For example, longing, regret, friendship, honor, worry. That person returns and the group interacts with him or her expressing that emotion, without using the actual word. The person who was chosen has to guess and name the emotion. This usually leads to a cathartic experience via the use of that emotion due to the enabling environment.

Our participants love these exercises. They encourage expression and develop empathy.

For a closing exercise, repeat the emotions that were used in this session and have the participants finish the sentence:

- "I feel frustrated when . . ."
- "When I feel frustrated . . ."
- "I feel cheerful when . . ."

- "When I feel cheerful . . ."
- "I feel angry when . . ."
- "When I am angry . . ."
- "Others are angry at me, when . . ."
- "I feel lonely when . . ."
- "When I feel lonely . . ."
- "I am disappointed when . . ."
- "When I am disappointed . . ."
- "Others are disappointed at me, when . . ."
- "I am happy when . . ."
- "When I am happy . . ."
- "I am happy with myself when . . ."
- "I am proud of . . ."
- "Others are proud of me when . . ."
- Continue with any other emotion on the list.

Suggestion: Whenever someone tells a personal story, it is always helpful to ask what emotions were felt in this incident. I always have my emotion cards with me in my basket.

Drama Games

Simple Improvisations

We discover that our group members love doing improvisations. These are a few of the openers for some of them. I call them rehearsals for possible situations that could arise. Their responses are very helpful and realistic.

The participants take turns playing the roles and reversing roles.

The following are the openers:

"Hi Mom . . . Hi dad . . ."

- "We can't come see you this week. We are too busy."
- "We came to tell you that we are moving to another city, country etc."
- "We want you to go to a nursing home."
- "We want you to go to Melabev."

Next situation:

- "There is a man outside who refuses to come in. What can you say to him to invite him to join our group?"

Followed by:

- You are sitting with your doctor. He tells you: "You need to use a walker."

Or he tells you:

- "You can no longer eat sugar."

The participants role-play the doctor and themselves with lots of role reversals with our young amazing volunteer, Michal. Each time, we try a few different approaches to dealing with these issues and conflicts. They acquire and absorb the options. Eventually, *they* suggest more personal situations for improvisations.

I am always surprised at how adept the participants are in playing roles that are fiction. They enjoy the *aesthetic distance* of drama games and improvisations. This is not necessarily about me. It is about anyone. I am portraying someone else. It is safe and it is fun.

The favorite improvisation is a situation between two people where the words: "no", "not" and "never" are forbidden. I start with a situation that is safe and not risky.

- One person is the sales person at an ice cream store. He has all the flavors. (My scarves of all colors represent these flavors) He is out of chocolate. The second person has come to purchase a delicious scrumptious ice cream cone on a very hot day. She or he likes only chocolate.

Open with: "Let's see what happens between you when you cannot speak in the negative." As soon as one person says no, someone else takes his or her place. This facilitates and encourages more participation and also has a side benefit of practicing positive communication.

After this situation which is not risky nor personal, slowly introduce scenarios where they can identify with the players.

- Your doctor, tells you to avoid sugar completely. You LOVE cake! You are not allowed to say "no". Let's see and hear how you and your doctor might discuss this.
- A scene between you and your aide. You tell him or her to buy you a box of cookies at the supermarket. The aide cannot do this because of your special diet restrictions. Let's hear the conversation without the word "no".

When we do not say "no", we hear options and explanations. There is sincere constructive communication. The interaction is not aggressive and is much more pleasant.

Ask the participants to think of situations where the communication will be more effective, precise and pleasant without the word NO. This is the most important part of the session. Through these improvisations, we can get a glimpse into the world of our participants and the issues and predicaments they are dealing with in their here and now. They get a chance to share their frustrations, fears and foibles.

Another very successful and easy game:

Identify the Changes

- Someone leaves the room. We make a few changes. She or he comes back into the room and has to notice these changes.

Here are a few simple examples:

- Have two people change seats.
- Two people exchange a piece of clothing; a scarf, necklace, cap, sweater.
- One woman removes one earring.
- One man removes his shoes.

These games work with any group aged 4–100.

The people who are involved in the change, experience *grandiosity*. They feel special. They know everyone is focused on them. The person who has to find what we changed, is also the center of attention and has to be alert and focused. The entire group has to remember what changes were made. Everyone's cognition level is stimulated and elevated. Participants seem to grow internally in this exercise. I can feel it as they show their joy with their bodies. It is especially exciting to see who volunteers to be the next person to leave the room and face this challenge. This is the challenge group and the participants are not threatened by the challenge but rather stimulated and inspired to try something new in a fun-loving environment. What's more, this is a memory game for a group of people who *cannot remember*!

This is the challenge group and the participants are not threatened by the challenge but rather stimulated and inspired to try something new in a fun-loving environment.

Summary of Practical Applications

- There are many psychodrama tools and methods such as working with a partner in the drama gift shop, using puppets, emotion exercises where the members have to guess what emotion is being expressed, drama games and improvisations related to the daily lives of the participants. They can all be applied to this population to induce comfort, a deep sense of belonging and identification.

- Emotion exercises can raise awareness of the vast array of emotions in daily experience and interactions and help participants gain tools and motivation to function emotionally with more control and confidence. All of this leads to releasing and sharing what is buried deep inside.
- Whenever someone tells a personal story, it is always helpful to ask what emotions were felt in this incident
- By writing a note, without signing it, on a subject that might be awkward or too exposing, folding it and placing it in an impressive hat or any other receptacle. The "Hat of Fear" is a method that provides anonymity which enables freedom of expression.
- Working with this interactive approach generates authentic expression and revelation, and the sharing of insights which also promotes a change in self-image.
- Creating a facilitative atmosphere through drama games helps overcome loneliness.
- Using techniques such as guessing what emotions are being acted out or having the participants role-play the doctor or the aide and themselves with lots of role reversals induces bonding, social-cohesion and new insights.
- Being playful is a magnet and distracts the participants from their aches and frustrations.

Part IV

Observing the Process

A Selection of Documented Sessions

Sharing My Rationale

I am now going to proceed with detailed documentation of many moving sessions that might give you, the reader, triggers, insights and options for activities and subjects to pursue with the people under your care or with your relatives and friends. We all recognize that these are people who need stimulation in order to function better in their daily routines. They spend a few hours a day at the Day Care Center. But what happens to their cognition when they are at home? Even though their family members might be available to supply their physical needs, these people, who are suffering from various forms of dementia, basically have a lonely existence at home. They are afraid to make mistakes. It is easier to simply withdraw and close their eyes, ears and minds. These sessions include wake-up exercises that will induce involvement and self-efficacy. In these psychodrama enactments, the players can actually make mistakes and learn how to correct them with a new confidence and vitality.

The following documentation of sessions contains gems of authentic expressions filled with wisdom, charm, insight and dignity. It is my hope that they will help readers understand the dilemmas, conflicts, frustrations, joys, achievements – and the potential of this population. These sessions are written in the first person about what I did as the group leader. My hope is that after reading these procedures, you will adapt them to your needs.

Aside from constantly trusting the process, one main rationale behind the subjects I choose to bring to our sessions is: what themes will stimulate expression, self-esteem and social cohesion? Over the course of these six years, we have covered almost everything related to their lives. As mentioned earlier, there were times that the subject matter was based on the here and now. At other times, they were connected to the calendar, current events near and far, or emotions that needed therapy. Or even something just for fun.

DOI: 10.4324/9781003321705-4

I also used news about a member of the group, an announcement such as a grandchild getting married. Another subject could be something light and fun, or a sensitive, serious or distracting issue.

These illustrations, with the responses of this group, will give you inside views of the needs of older adults, the desires of the people who are suffering from various forms of dementia. When you read the details, you will be more sensitive to their pain, passion, pride and prudence.

In the documentation of these sessions, genuine gems of truth leap off the page. They are filled with sensitivity, spontaneity and a desire for quality lives filled with communication and understanding.

In his book, Covenant and Conversation, Deuteronomy (2019), Rabbi Jonathan Sacks, of blessed memory, talks about the importance of memory in a completely different context. However, some of his sentences made me think of the importance of finding exercises that will help our population recall and remember. Sentences like, "We are what we remember." "The loss of memory is experienced as a total loss of identity." Yes, this is the rationale for everything we do in our circle of trust. We help the participants realize, know and appreciate who they are. Rabbi Sacks further strengthens the goals and the methods of drama when he quotes Alasdair MacIntyre's (2007) book, *After Virtue*, (University of Notre Dame Press) in talking about the importance of narrative to the moral life, "Man, in his actions and practice, as well as in his fictions, is essentially a story-telling animal." Rabbi Sacks explains, "It is through narrative that we begin to learn who we are and how we are called on to behave" (Sacks, 2019, p. 223–225).

Using a True Story as a Trigger

I walk into the room. Twenty wonderful people are sitting in a circle. You can see their eagerness and positive anticipation. There is an aura of hope and promise in the air. They are waiting to hear what subject we are going to warm up with. This passivity may come from their reluctance to initiate, or it may be the result of the various physical or mental constraints brought on by old age or dementia.

Sometimes I bring in a true story from my life. I may relate to current events or seasonal issues. Occasionally, the subject for our session will evolve during the *checking in* – when everyone simply tells us how they are doing or relates something about their week or morning, or simply something nice or new that they want to share with us. This can be developed through action, in our session. At other times the group counselor will advise me of a new issue that needs to be addressed. It is all very natural and comfortable for everyone including me. This atmosphere is contagious and helps to stimulate inclusion and responsiveness. For example, I open up the session by telling them a true story:

Yesterday, my husband got a phone call from a very wealthy relative in New Jersey. He even has a private airplane! He just turned eighty and he heard that you can buy stem cells and have them injected into your body and that will help you stay young. My husband, a medical researcher, told his relative that he did not recommend this procedure.

I then put our *empty chair* out in front of them and say:

I am inviting this cousin to come and sit in this chair. Let's imagine that he is right here in front of us all, nice and comfortable. We know we can do this in psychodrama. Now, because you are all so wise, I would like you to give him advice from your life experience. Here he is. Talk to him. You have so much to share. Let's hear.

I start because I have found that it helps the group to hear examples from me. I say to the *empty chair*, "Be creative. Try something new." This gets the ball rolling.

Pauline: "Give your money to charity. It will make you feel good."

I stand behind Pauline and say what I think she is feeling but not saying. We call this "being a double".

Double: *When we feel good about our actions, we feel young.*
Martin: "Keep busy."
Brian: "I get my wife to yell at me."
Jake: "Songs, music. Songs that you love. Sing, listen to music."
Lila: "Read a few newspapers."

She tells the story of how she read about Israel's space capsule, Bereshit. Israel is the fourth country in the world with such an amazing achievement. And then she told her daughter the news. It turned out that her daughter was involved in this project.

Double: *Keep informed so that you are in the know and are interested and interesting. It helps you connect with others in many ways. Connecting through being informed.*

Lila loves this double. It reminds her that she does have a brain and she actually does use it. Thanks to this exercise, she is able to share this and feel informed and proud. She has regained a sense of dignity which she so desperately needs.

Manny: "I like to solve problems. If something is wrong, fix it. If you can."
Double: *This empowers me. I have always been very good at fixing things.*

Manny nods affirmatively.

Martin:	"Try to eat right. Don't eat too much. Don't eat heavy foods. Watch your weight. Get advice from a good dietician."
Herbie:	"I enjoy reading scientific and technical journals."
Susan:	"Play with the kids."
Debra:	"Get a good night's sleep."
Janet:	"You are only as old as you feel."
Pauline:	"Appreciate what you have."
Martin:	"Do what you can, as much as you can."
Double:	*"Take advantage of today. You don't know what tomorrow will bring."*

The eating message from Manny is spontaneously opened up into a short vignette where Manny, who suffers from diabetes and is over-weight, admits that his wife is very strict with him. At night he sneaks food from the kitchen. I ask him to talk to the food and tell the food why he cannot touch it. He ends up allowing himself a small piece of choco-late. I am not sure this scene helped Manny but it did illustrate for all the others the effects of poor eating habits. It also put him in the limelight. He needs this *grandiosity*. His declining situation leaves him filled with humiliation. The food gives him the satisfaction he is seeking.

This was a very empowering session. The participants deal daily with their challenges, inadequacies, ailments, difficulties, as well as fears of further deterioration of their cognition. In this exercise with the *empty chair*, they were talking to someone who was trying to bypass the chal-lenges these people face daily. Through psychodrama, they can find their strengths and strategies for coping.

To close the session, I do a double for the wealthy relative who is "sit-ting" in the *empty chair*, and I say, *"I wish I had the strength to accept, and enjoy what I CAN do and be in a group like this where I could appreciate the joys of aging like all of you."*

In this session, we are able to ascertain that the participants are comfortable talking about the most personal issues. I spontaneously put an imaginary genie in the *empty chair* and, with a wink, ask them what they would, nevertheless, like to get from the genie that would help them feel and stay young. I tell them, "Why not take advantage of drama? Let's pretend this genie is here listening to your requests. It's always fun to make a wish." One man admits that even though he is 91, he needs sex and his wife won't cooperate. The people in the group understand his need – especially the other men. He feels validated and he feels young.

Lionel wants to take a cruise through the Panama Canal. Another woman asks her grandchildren to visit more often. Our participants feel safe in asking the genie for what they need. These are actually realistic requests. Their needs are given a strong, healthy voice.

Resilience

I decide to talk about an invaluable attribute for coping: resilience. So, I put this question to the group, "What is *bouncing back* for you?" We sculpt the word "resilience" with the colored scarves (Image 4.1). Again, they receive options, identification with others in the group and validation. So, do I!

Lilly: willpower (mild pink)
Avi: reframing (gold, blue and green)
Benjy: making choices (orange)
Harvey: finding a new direction (red)
Jacob: compromise (burgundy)
Deena: being sensible (as usual, purple)
Pauline: when my husband has a good day, coping (royal blue)
Barbara: accepting criticism constructively and not speaking back (sunny yellow)
Rosie: acceptance (white)
Lionel: creativity (green)

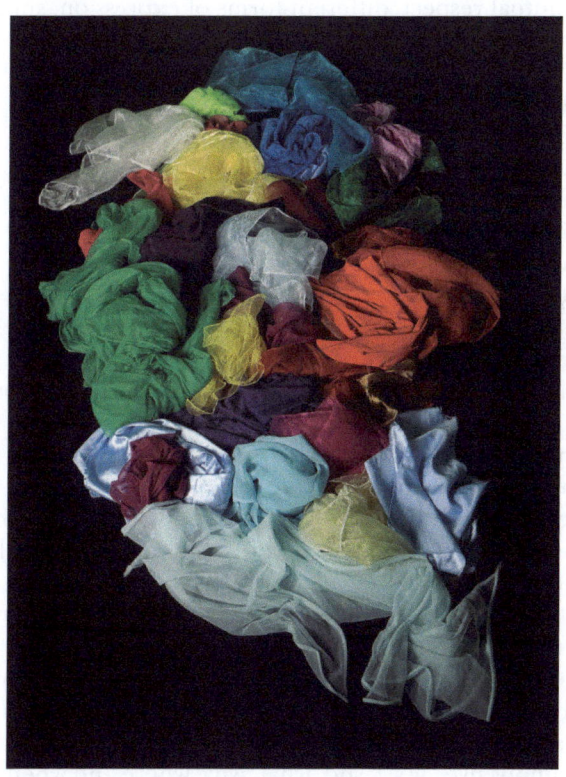

Image 4.1

We all look at this many-faceted depiction of resilience sculpted by the group. Yes, there are various ways to cope, to bounce back, to accept, to change, to move on. The participants are invited to share their stories. We hear stories from the past and the present and gain the strength we need for the future.

Theme – LOVE. Technique: Imaginary Photo Albums

I say, "Today our subject is LOVE." That certainly gets their attention!

Warm-up

I ask the group: When you think of LOVE, show me how you look?

(It is interesting to note differences in gender response.) In this particular group, the words flow but the ability to act out what they are saying and *show* us is much more challenging. However, their eyes are filled with the essence of these following descriptions of love.

Barbara:	hugging, holding, touching, togetherness
Moe:	mutual respect, different forms of expression, snuggling
Martin:	showing through giving
Pauline:	appreciation, being thankful, comforting
Hannah:	happiness
Me:	commitment, trust, loyalty, a memory
Zeev:	commitment, everyone loves their mother, even if she is a nag.
Brian:	let's go to bed
Monica:	warmth
Lionel:	unconditional

I now proceed with the session using the technique of Imaginary Photo Albums. Using these imaginary albums helps the group retrieve memories and relive emotional experiences that raise their self-esteem and awareness. This is a method that always works. Here is a detailed, well-documented illustration.

I say: "Let's imagine that you can open up your photo albums. Let's wipe off the dust from the album covers. Open up a few until you find a photo that depicts love."

In order to get this going, I describe a picture of my father looking at me, with tender loving eyes, at my wedding.

I continue, "When you find the perfect photo, think to yourself: Who is in the photo? What is happening? Why was it photographed? When was this photo taken? Where is the location?"

Yes, the famous five "w's": who, what, why, where and when. I tell them that reporters always have to make sure they include answers to all five when they write about an event. Now I begin a short exercise in *guided imagery* in order to help them connect and concentrate. I know I will be repeating instructions, but for this group, it is necessary. I continue, addressing the group as a whole:

> You are now reporting on an important part of your life. Let's all close our eyes. I am also going to close my eyes. You don't have to, if it is not comfortable for you, but it helps. Now go to the album you selected. Open it. Find that fabulous photo and answer the five "w's". Also think about: Where is this photo taking place? Who else is in the photo? What are you wearing in this photo? Who took the photo? Why did this moment deserve to be photographed? What time of day is it? What is your age here?

Enough warm up. We are ready to enact this subject. I guide them to think of the photo that captures love and then some of the participants tell us a bit about the photograph they chose. I then ask: "Now, who wants to see their photo come alive? We can do it here and now and recapture our past." This works. They are ready for action!

First enactment: The photograph is presented by **Martin**. In his photo, he and his wife are standing in their backyard by their fruit trees. Martin is the director and does the casting. This is a perfect example of empowerment. He picks one volunteer to play him and another to play his wife. We then stage the photo of Martin and his loving wife. His arm is around her and he is holding her close to his side. They are in their backyard in New York. We could all imagine seeing their children. They are all there. Martin and his wife are enjoying watching the children playing together, before they sit down to eat their barbeque lunch. You could feel his love for his wife, who passed away over ten years ago. And since he is directing this creation, he has the person playing his wife look at the person playing him with deep love. He directs the scene insistently until it is perfect in his eyes. He is able to look at this depiction and recall how much love there was in his marriage, within his family, and in their home. It is a remarkably poignant scene.

We can see this classic example of *mirroring* when Martin looks at the scene he has directed, and blurts out, "Our home was filled with warmth and love. We did not have to go anywhere to feel this joy." He then plays himself. The staff helps him to stand. He tells his wife how much he loved her.

After this vignette, the sharing around the group is filled with simple stories of the security of home, backyards, barbeques. . . . It illuminates their lives with meaning. In the sharing after an enactment the participants talk about how they connected to the scene in their personal lives. They share the ways in which it touched them emotionally and what memories came up for them. We hear a lot of expressions of love, caring and good times.

Barbara is next. The photo is of her and her two granddaughters, sitting together in the garden of her son's home where she has an apartment downstairs. The photo is staged. The volunteers help Barbara to our "stage" where she directs them on how to set up the scene.

She is the central character in this scene and she loves it. This is a perfect example of *grandiosity*.

Barbara: "It's okay in the garden. It's natural." She is in the middle and two volunteers playing her 15-year-old and 16-year-old granddaughters are sitting on both sides of her and leaning their heads on her shoulders.

"It feels so nice. When there is contact and touch between them and me, I'm feeling warm. They love me."

Me: "What do you want to say to them as they sit with you like this?"
Barbara: "I'm so glad when you show me love. It makes me feel so nice."
Me: "Give this picture of you and your granddaughters a name."
Barbara: "Loveable."

The memories that are evoked are so vivid and authentic.

Lionel: "I always photograph the people I love."

Next comes **Adrienne**. She asks us to stage a picture of her and her four sons and one daughter at a wedding. They are all standing behind her.

Adrienne: "Always my babies!"
Deena: "This brings up memories. Sad that my husband is not here to share them."

Now it's **Moe:** "I saw my wife on the stage at Junior High School. She was fourteen. I was sixteen. (He was actually 98 when he said this!) I liked the way she presented herself. She was very pretty, even though she wore glasses. Men don't usually make passes at girls with glasses."

The memories are flowing. The comments are sharp and precise and filled with ardor and humor. These comments are what Moreno called *sharing*.

Benjy: (His cognition is deteriorating rapidly. It is so nice to hear him retrieve information that he can share with us and find the words to express himself. This is a man who was having difficulty putting together a few words and this stimulus miraculously aroused him to tell an entire story! Sadly, this did not prove to be a permanent change.)

"My parents got married three times! They were in a concentration camp and had planned to marry as soon as they were released from the camp. An edict went out, stating that all single men would be killed the following day. They were married that night. The second time, they were in Prague. They got their papers together and got married. The third time was when they came to the U.S.A."

Pauline: "My first husband died in a car accident. My second husband – well, that was a big love story that lasted fifty years! I was on a pedestal so high, I got nose bleeds."

The session is over but love is in the air.

I have used this technique of photos at other sessions. I would ask for scenes for our album of Happy Moments filled with laughter and joy. Yes, we have those too. We have made imaginary photo albums from holidays, the different seasons, events in their lives – even their Bar Mitzvas. They are all as moving as this session.

The Telephone Technique

This is a good opportunity to explain a basic term in psychodrama – Moreno's term *tele* (pronounced tay-lay). With this group, it can be referring to a non-verbal communication between two people, a deep rapport between two people, or a very empathic communication that leads to a deep connection. We experience this amazing connection when I take up the role of a *double* and say what I think they are feeling but not saying, or when they do deep, honest sharing after a short psychodrama enactment. This deep connection is touching and very meaningful. Achieving *tele* is a great accomplishment in a group where people are so challenged cognitively. I certainly have no intentions of using *tele* the way it is used in psychodrama groups *sociometrically*. I am mostly interested in helping our participants connect to themselves and their innermost feelings and to one another. There is a detailed elaboration on this important term in the Glossary of Terms and Elaborations.

Tele is used in the old-fashioned way in this session when I place an old-fashioned *tele*phone on our *empty chair* in the center of our inimitable circle. We do not achieve Moreno's *tele*, but we do accomplish deep and authentic expression. I do not know what will develop but, I know there will be a special communication. Moreno would approve.

This session proceeds as follows: I place an authentic, old-fashioned dial telephone on a chair in the center of the circle. I tell them: "In psychodrama, we can make almost anything happen. We can call anyone we want with this telephone. Just dial and tell the person whatever it is you need to say to them. Take advantage of this incredible opportunity to express yourself."

Everyone in the staff is shocked when Deena responds. Aged 94, she invariably shies away from expressing herself and says just two words, "*oy vey*". This "*oy vey*" receives the *double*, "*Oh I don't know what to say, no-one believes me. I am too old to express myself. I don't want to say something stupid. Maybe I didn't understand your direction.*"

So many expressions of a lack of confidence. But today we are pleasantly surprised because she announces, with ease and confidence as if a magnet had pulled her to the phone. "I want the phone. I want to call my son who died six months ago."

Me: "What's his name?"
Deena: "Moe."

And she continues it as if there is no one in the room listening. She goes right to it.

"We miss you. We miss the jokes that you told us. We love you and all the children you left us."

Brian, aged 91, is so moved by this endearing authentic expression of love, that he spontaneously gets out of his seat, walks over to her and kisses her on the forehead and says, "You are not alone darling."

I ask her, "How do you feel now?"

Deena: (with the most beautiful sweet smile) "A little bit better."

I then say, "We just experienced true love." Deena is feeling validated, from this instance of *tele* with Brian. This is so therapeutic for a woman suffering from paranoia.

Everyone is feeling comfortable with this telephone being passed around from the center of our circle. And maybe this is actually what Moreno was referring to with the word *tele* – communication that is so deep.

Then, **Lionel,** aged 73, takes the phone. It all pours out, with incredible emotion!

> Why don't you answer when I call? Are you embarrassed that you still owe us the money? We're coming on a cruise, via Panama. (Yes, that cruise that he had wished for the week before.) We're coming to collect it. You're still not doing what I told you. Be a singer. You've got a wonderful voice. I'm bloody disgusted with your children. They've all come here and none got in touch with me.

To the group while holding the receiver in his hand and covering it at the same time. "This is my wife's brother. He lost his house. He messed up his life. He should return to his family in Israel, but he is too ashamed."

I then ask him, "If you could really speak to him, would you say everything you just said?"

Lionel, "He doesn't answer the phone."

Me:	"You really want this cruise."
Lionel:	"I am looking into a trip to L.A. via the Panama Canal. I'm trying to exhibit my artwork, on the ship, to pay for the trip."
Double:	*I've got to do this now, while I can. I'm trying all sorts of ways to make it work.*

Next, **Lila** takes the phone. Aged 87, hers is a practical request. She is cutting through the frustration of bureaucracy by using our phone to ask the army a few questions pertaining to her granddaughter. She wants them to allow her to go to her cousin's wedding in the United States. We open this into a vignette and again meet her granddaughter, Lila loves *role-playing* this young very smart, studious and ambitious granddaughter.

Zeev, aged 87, who falls asleep a lot in our sessions, uses the phone to call his wife to tell her exactly what he wants to eat for dinner. He is awake and alert, involved and hungry.

Then **Brian** lets his heart talk, via the phone, to his two brothers who have been gone quite a long time. It is heart-wrenching to hear his pain, remorse, love and longing. It is a catharsis that helps him realize how much love is in his heart.

There are other phone calls that are so fluid and real that they prompt **Moe**, aged 98, who has come just for the psychodrama session, to say: "I want to call my daughter, but| I don't remember her phone number!!! Is this a real phone?" He was so convinced that there was someone at the other end of the line listening to every word, that he believed these were two-way conversations. He did not understand how they reached the person so quickly! This led him to share how he actually talks to his daughter and grandchildren every day on Skype.

Barbara, aged 94, was warmed up and took the phone and announced "I'm going to call my husband who passed away sixteen years ago.

I just want to tell you I love you and miss you. I miss all the good times we had together – all the travelling. You were always so healthy."

I then very impulsively asked for her permission to talk to him. She handed me the phone.

"Hi", I say. "Your wife comes here to Melabev. She dresses so nicely. She doesn't look her age at all."

Barbara, "And tell him I lost fifteen kilos. He didn't like fat ladies."

I repeat that message to him and Barbara is so pleased with herself.

Our action then turns to the subject of the need to communicate. Martin states that he prefers face-to-face communication, whenever it is possible. He understands the *surplus reality* of our phone conversation. We role-play

his conversations with his grandsons who are no longer religiously obser-
vant yet, who knows, they might return to tradition. He lets them know
that he is proud of their basic values. This is a recurring theme for Martin.
Our sessions help him vent his frustration with his grandsons leaving the
religious way of life and examine his feelings about their choices.

Yes, we can have empathy and deep communication between people
with various forms and degrees of dementia.

> Yes, we can have empathy and deep communication between peo-
> ple with various forms and degrees of dementia.

Seeing Your Name in Action

As we progress, I am brave and try more complicated activities.

For example, I hand out paper and pencils and boards to lean on and
I say, "Write the letters of your name and give an adjective about yourself
for each letter." I give them an example with the letters of my name using
a lot of adjectives that are candid and revealing, in order to demonstrate
the multitude of options and encourage transparency.

- T = truthful, talkative, temperamental
- Z = zany
- I = intuitive, impulsive
- P = pleasing, perfectionist, placating
- P = performer, proud, poetic
- I = imaginative, interesting

We then do this exercise with one of our volunteers to further demonstrate.

These revealing examples encourage the participants to write sincerely
about themselves. I also let them know that if anyone needs help in writing, they can dictate to our staff and volunteers. I continue, "Let's hear
what you have written." Everyone reads their composition (*grandiosity*). The
audience enjoys listening to one another.

After hearing what they wrote, which is very moving, I then ask for a volunteer or choose an appropriate *protagonist*. I say, "Let's SEE your name. You
will be the director of this production (empowerment). First, as the director,
you do the casting. Who in the group can you cast to depict each descriptive
adjective for each letter?" After our session with photo albums, this group is
familiar with this terminology and even adept at casting and directing.

Adrienne volunteers with gusto. She picks the people for each letter.
They are called *auxiliary egos* in the psychodrama language. We then
build a vignette out of this group of actors. The *protagonist*, Adrienne,

gives each *auxiliary ego*, who is depicting an adjective, a typical pose or movement and a characteristic sentence.

Adrienne picks, excuse me, casts, someone to be her. This person is actually another form of what, in psychodrama, we call a *double*. As the director, she stages and places all of the actors (*auxiliary egos*) in relation to the person depicting her and, as a result, has an opportunity to look at this scene from the outside and receive *mirroring* in action. I then ask Adrienne, the protagonist, if and how she would like to change this detailed self-portrait.

In order to avoid divulging the actual name of the person who did this exercise, I will elaborate with only three letters in her name. Adrienne is the fictional name of the person who volunteered to bring her name to an action. I will elaborate on three letters from her name; A.I.N.

Adrienne reads out the adjectives she has just written for the letters in her name and then selects people in the group who remind her of these traits. All of these participants now have the experience of being auxiliary egos and Adrienne is proudly the casting director.

*A*drie*n*ne is

A

Adventurous = Martin
Able = David
Anti-disestablishment = Jake
Amicable = Herbie
Aware = Jacob

I

Interesting = Moe
Involved = Pauline
Individual = Debra

N

Nice and normal = Yocheved

Adrienne does a very precise casting. She selects the people from the group who are really fine examples of the traits they would be portraying in this psychodrama exercise. She then gives each person their text and an appropriate action and actually goes about staging them on our improvised stage at the front of the room. We are getting an action that has been written, casted and directed by our very own Adrienne. She tells them where and how to stand or sit. She gives their hands and bodies proper motions and gives them their text. This is empowering and inclusive. A very large number of people from the group are participating. It is almost a phenomenon. That is why I am describing it in such detail.

- **Martin**, as adventurous: "I am always there and everywhere."
- **David**, as able: "To help and listen to others."
- **Jake**, as anti-disestablishment: "It's not what you want."
- **Jacob**, as aware: "I always know what is going on around me by looking at people and noticing their mood changes."
- **Herbie,** as amicable: Adrienne instructs him to just simply smile.
- **Moe**, as interesting: "I have an interesting story to share."
- **Dorothy**, as individual: (Adrienne confesses) "I always got punished in school because I always laughed last. I will get the last laugh."
- **Yocheved**, as nice and normal: "Just being myself."

I ask Adrienne if this is a true and accurate action portrait of herself. She is very certain that it is. Her face is glowing. This is enough for one session.

Many times, when I do this exercise, I ask the person who is the combination of protagonist, scriptwriter and director if there is anything they would like to stage differently, remove or add. The results are always revealing and truthful. In this case, Adrienne got an enormous amount of satisfaction from portraying herself inside and out. It is a shame she did not remember this action at our next session. Most of these participants hardly remembered. We have learned to live with that fact. We did, however, have a very consequential production. At this moment, we could add theatre to our repertoire of activities. We have a stage. We have actors, a director, texts and movement; again – the Theatre of Truth!

The Use of Masks – Examples of Flexibility

You have just read accounts of a few sessions that our group responded to easily. It is so nice to write up these sessions and leave you with the impression that everything works. But, believe me, it is not so simple. I would like to discuss what we can do when the session isn't working as planned. This happens often. Now *I* am dealing with challenge!

First, analyze the reason that the group is not responding – but quickly and coolly. Is it not working because your directions are not clear, too complicated, or too close for comfort? Or, is it not working because the participants simply are not capable of doing what you planned? There is nothing wrong with saying, okay, this is not working, let's try something else, or to just smoothly move on to something similar that they *can* handle. No fuss. I would like to share one of those days with you.

I walk in with an array of beautiful masks. (See photo, in PART IV Sharing From My Process With Adolescents) I have a feeling this might not work, but I give it a try because the outcome can be transformative. Working with masks might be too difficult for most of them. Here is a description of the session.

In honor of the Jewish holiday of Purim, where masks and costumes are a major highlight of the holiday celebration. I place some beautiful character masks in the center of the circle, on the floor. I ask the participants to select a mask without revealing their choice to the group. I then ask them to concentrate on the mask of their choice and create a character. Once they connect to the character they are creating, I tell them to give it a name, address, date of birth, profession, and then we can guess which mask they are thinking of. I am so focused on my plans that I am not understanding that I have already lost most of the participants.

I am so focused on my plans that I am not understanding that I have already lost most of the participants.

I continue confidently that next they would be given the mask of their choice to wear. They would become the person they had just created. We would then see if wearing the mask and becoming someone else changes their body language and their way of speaking. These were my expectations!

I've done this exercise with many other groups and the results are always interesting and revealing and enjoyable for everyone. I want to recapture the magic of the session when I did this exercise with a drama therapy group of eighth graders and a non-verbal girl found her voice and expressed herself freely and openly. I came in on this day with high hopes and great expectations.

Only one person in the Melabev group, Lionel, is able to do this. It is definitely worth it to see him become a gorgeous young girl. He was so happy! But that is it. I then immediately change my plans and ask the staff to do this exercise and the people in the group can simply interview the characters the staff creates. We do not get the anticipated results but it does lead to expression in front of the group. This is no minor accomplishment for them and maybe I'll think of a different way to present this exercise more simply by letting them simply put on the masks and see themselves and one another. This way they can enjoy the magic in the transformation. That's enough!

I then spontaneously use the inspiration of this demonstration and ask each of them, if you could be someone else for a day, or even an hour, who would you want to be? This they *can* do and their responses evoke stories and the sharing of experiences.

Some of the participants want to be themselves at different stages of their life. Memories are recalled and stories are told. Others want to be: Toscanini, Sid Caesar, the Hunchback of Notre Dame, The Count of Monte Cristo and Einstein. I ask them what they would like to take from the characters they selected and their responses are totally appropriate and satisfying and cathartic.

This improvised exercise has come about naturally, without a fuss, and everyone is happy with the way the masks are used as an introduction to the joys of being someone else on a holiday that is filled with masquerading. What evolved as a result of the initial "failure" has turned out to be a much more appropriate exercise for this group. If necessity is the mother of invention, then flexibility is the father of creativity.

If necessity is the mother of invention, then flexibility is the father of creativity

---

I would like to share another aspect of flexibility. When I try to do role reversals with this population, some of the group members are incapable of being the other person, so I play the other person and ask them to give me my text in the role I am playing for them. When the volunteers are capable and free, I ask them to be the *auxiliary ego* and to implement the role reversal. This way, I can conduct the enactment more effectively. I am fortunate to have staff and volunteers in the room during our sessions. One volunteer who joined us in my second year with this group, Michal, actually studied psychodrama. She is always exactly what is needed in the role reversals. I am fortunate to have such a spontaneous sensitive professional *auxiliary ego*. She is devoted and empathic to our participants: her instincts guide her to know what to say and exactly how to say it. Her account of her experience with this group appears in PART VIII, the section called "Sharing From Members of Our Staff". The only participants who could play roles in someone else's vignette are Avi and Lionel.

The staff and volunteers are full participants in all the exercises so that the group will not feel that they have an audience. The staff is open, ready to be exposed and express themselves honestly. One volunteer is in her eighties. This transparency also encourages the participants to express themselves freely. Sometimes the staff is busy with technical aspects of the group (like giving someone a drink or escorting them to the bathroom) and I have to do all the action myself. My openness with them is an invitation for them to share. It is vital for the leader or facilitator in this group process, to not be distant or reticent.

Stories From Periods in Our Lives

It is easier for this population to retrieve memories from their past. For a series of sessions, we recounted memories from the decades of our lives.

From 0 to 10: growing up, starting school.

From 11 to 20: adolescence, teenage adventures and mishaps

From 20 to 30: falling in love, getting married, becoming young parents.

From 30 to 40: building homes, dealing with family dynamics and expanding careers.

From 40 to 60: remembering our first child's wedding, dealing with in-laws or grandchildren. (Everyone in this group had children.)

I am not going to expand upon the responses to this theme, as this is not a book of biographies. It is a very significant subject for this population and should be in your repertoire when working with older adults and people who are dealing with dementia. Actually, this is a meaningful theme for any adult group. Everyone loves to go down memory lane and recall stories from the past. Robert Landy in, *Drama Therapy*, p. 224, sums it up poignantly:

For the drama to be more deeply therapeutic, the therapist must be willing to help his clients review their lives to discover a sense of purposefulness to uncover some of the guilt and confusion caused by social circumstances as well as personal choice and to move toward death, not with a sense of despair and regret, but with dignity and wisdom.

I do a short *guided imag*ery to connect the participants to their histories and if they are having trouble, I tell a brief story from my own life. This is a good trigger for them. The stories bring smiles, laughter, and a lot of connecting. We hear words like stoopball and expressions like playing in the gutter. Memories of families, friendships, naivete and innocence and many stories of hardship are shared. It is obvious that they are now feeling comfortable with one another and with themselves. They delight in remembering their achievements, their relationships. There is an energy of pride in our circle of story-telling and trust. They also discover a lot more things that they have in common.

I am always impressed at the respect they have for each other. They do not interrupt when someone is telling their story. They listen. They respond. They care. We all *see* it. We all *feel* it: the staff, myself and the participants.

On the other hand, some of the best sessions are the ones where we deal directly with the here and now. For example, at the end of June, when we are experiencing a severe heat wave, I conduct the session accordingly and focus on summer heat.

Summertime

Warm-up:
  When the weather is very hot, I . . .

- Water the plants.
- Take a shower.
- Make sure there is water for dogs and cats.
- Take off as much clothing as possible.
- I change my clothes and sit by a fan.
- Put on the air conditioner.
- I sweat.
- I wilt.
- I suffer.
- I drink, everyone should drink at least six to eight glasses a day.
- I drink and play with the garden hose.
- I find a place that is cooler.
- I try to stay inside.
- I distract myself from the heat.
- I have an argument with my son. My son is never hot. I am always sweating. (Her unmarried son lives with her.)
- I'm fine. It doesn't bother me.

Speaking to the group is not a simple task for all of the participants. Some of them respond easily. When the subject is connected to something they are experiencing in the here and now, the first few responses are a trigger for those who find it difficult to find the words and lack the confidence to speak up and express themselves. The man who says, "I drink and play with the garden hose", never initiates a comment yet here, it seems to just blurt out of his mouth. Thanks to the enabling environment, he is participating with ease and comfort. He feels vital. He is alive! I am so happy for him.

This warm-up spontaneously opens into sharing memories from times past in the old country when it was hot outside.

Someone says, "I used to tell my husband, let's go to (an air conditioned) department store and sit in the shoe department and then have milk shakes for dinner at the soda-fountain."

When beginning a sentence with the words, "I remember" quick responses follow.

- We went to the beach.
- We used to burst the tar bubbles from the road.
- The ice cream truck with music would come to our street. I remember the merry jingle of the music.
- Watermelon, Italian ices, ice cream, snow cones.

- We went to a movie in an air-conditioned theater.
- Bungalows, up in the mountains, where you could jump into the pool or the lake in a minute.

All of these associations awake memories of good times in the summer that the participants share. It is always very effective to give them some *mirroring* – a technique where they can see themselves. This is done by asking them to think of how they would sculpt themselves in a typical summer pose. They can then choose one of the volunteers to role reverse and play themselves and other people in this summer picture, acting as *auxiliary egos*, when necessary. There are always volunteers in the room. Most of the volunteers are social work students doing their internship at our center. Sometimes, we succeed in choosing one of the more mobile participants to be an auxiliary ego and play a role.

Here are examples:

> "I am waving good-bye. I have a big smile on my face. It was too hot to stay in the city, so my parents sent me to summer camp. I loved it."
> "We also went away to the bungalow colony. My picture is carrying a suitcase."
> "Eating watermelon on the stoop"
> "Swimming"
> "Jumping into the water"
> "Staying with my grandparents"

In each case, they tell our volunteers exactly how to stand. They are the directors and sculptors of their "live" pictures. The *protagonist* tells the actors (*auxiliary egos*) what expression to have on their face, how to stand, where to place their hands. Then they give them a sentence to say. In each case, they look at the tableau of themselves in the summer, and give it a title. This is a form of *mirroring*, where they can see themselves brought to life in scenes from their past. All of these titled pictures revive lost memories. Again, there is empowerment in our circle of *sharing* through doing. There is an album of photos in our hearts. This is certainly enough for one session.

In another session on summertime, one year later, when the group was even more advanced and adept at using psychodrama in our sessions, I planned to develop a more sophisticated *action*.

Summertime Revisited

My original plan for this session:
"Think of a sentence that you would say in the summer?

Think of a sentence that you heard very often, in the summer.
Now think of what was your *double* when you said those typical
statements. What were you feeling but not saying?
For example: "I am so hot"
Double: *Why don't we have an air conditioner??*"
"Now let's see a typical summer scene. Let's build a panoramic picture
of summer activities." I found that these instructions were proving
too complicated for the participants. Here is another example of
flexibility and spontaneity in working with this group. This is a good
opportunity to describe what happens when you plan an activity and
you realize quite quickly that this particular group cannot comply.
Either they are physically limited or cognitively incapable. If you use
this opportunity to be flexible and spontaneous, the way that Moreno,
the father of psychodrama recommended, you can have a surprisingly
successful session. Here is the outcome of the revised session on
summertime. I had to start with an instruction that was simple.

Warm-up:

1.   "When you hear 'summertime' or simply the word 'summer', what is
     your first association?"

Daisy:	(a new member) Sun
Libby:	Coney Island
Mitch:	Sand in food
Martin:	Holy Holidays coming up
Herbie:	Hanging out
Deena:	Flowers
Lila:	(a new member who never speaks up but feels very comfortable with this subject) I love it.
Adrienne:	Trip to the beach, light clothing
Deena:	Getting lost
Manny:	Family gatherings
Martin:	Swimming in Peconic Bay.
Lionel:	Good evenings together
Daisy:	Grass
Lionel:	Sweating in Tel Aviv. Cool evenings in Jerusalem.
Geoffrey:	Pessimism (I purposely did not pursue this and waited to see how his attitude developed.)
Herbie:	Punch ball
Martin:	Going out in my uncle's boat.
Monica:	I would change my clothes and sit by a fan.
Brian:	Who remembers the iceman delivering big blocks of ice? Changing the water on the bottom of the ice box?

Daisy: Rowboats, transistor radios, sun mirror, beach balls. (She is actively enjoying the session and is far from embodying the word that she had given to describe herself at her first session: "morose"! She continues) camp, handball, golf, drive-in movies, camping.

The group is warmed up for the next exercise! I ask them: What are some of the sentences that typified your summer experiences? What do you remember saying often?

"But I don't have school tomorrow!"
"Oh, what a beautiful morning" (this was sung to us.)
"Let's do something."
"What time is it?"
"Let's go swimming."
"Ouch, my sunburn hurts."
"Where's the Noxzema?" (A cream that treats sunburns)
"Don't forget your bathing suit."
"Cut the grass"
"Rake the leaves"
"Move your butt, I'm falling out of the canoe."

They are in their summer setting and reliving their summer fun. Geoffrey, who had said, "pessimistic" adds this one-word sentence "Help!" upon which Barbara tells the story of how her husband was relaxing on the shore and she swam too far out and suddenly found herself in an undercurrent, fighting large waves. She waved her arms to get help but her husband thought she was saying hi. The lifeguard understood and he brought her in. She fainted when she touched solid ground. "That was a miracle. Thank God for miracles."

I ask who else almost drowned and we hear some interesting responses. I also share stories of the four to five times I almost drowned, including on my honeymoon! So important to encourage laughter.

The entire group was sharing experiences. Up until this point, the session proceeds as planned. I am sure they can continue as planned! As Moreno said, "Don't tell me, show me."

My next suggestion is, "Let's see some typical activities, poses and scenes of summertime. Who would like to show us?" No one volunteers. When this happens, I ask someone who I think is able and willing to "volunteer". I ask Lionel. He actually does a golf playing motion and elaborates on it. It is just what was needed. But, unfortunately, no one follows. It is too difficult for them. But something else does happen! Instead of scenes, we get something that they can do from the physical safety of their seats. We get songs and jingles from their childhood games. Before we know it, we are all singing and all the words that were not heard in many years, surface.

> *Cinderella dressed in yella,*
> *Went upstairs to kiss her fella.*
> *By mistake she kissed a snake,*
> *How many doctors will it take?*
> *1, 2, 3, 4, 5, 6, 7, 8, 9, etc.*
> *A – my name is Alice and my husband's name is Abe. We come from*
> *Alabama and we eat apples.*
> *Five, ten, fifteen, twenty, leave the rope empty.*

When this is sung, I take a volunteer and we pretend to be turning a jump rope and then more jump rope jingles surface. What follows immediately are the names of street games like Ringolevio, a tag game that was played on the streets of New York City. This, of course, brings more smiles of recognition to their faces. And then I ask a spontaneous question: "When you think of summer, who do you think of?" This ignites a new level of participation and connecting to their past. The participants not only introduce us to people in their lives, but also sing the songs and jingles they learned from them, and everyone joins in. It becomes an unplanned summer jam session.

It is common knowledge that music is very beneficial to Alzheimer patients. But, here, the music evolves from the context of the session. It is not artificially presented to them from the outside. It emerges from their associations, memories and connections. They work hard to remember the words and the actions and, as a group, because of the enabling environment, they succeed.

> *This old man, he played one.*
> *He played knick knack on my thumb.*
> *With a knick knack paddy wack,*
> *Give a dog a bone.*
> *This old man came rolling home.*

They are doing the motions up to four:

> *two – shoe,*
> *three – knee,*
> *four – door.*

There is a genuine excitement and participation. I know because I too am enjoying remembering and hearing all these childhood jingles.

Yes, true – I had planned that session with doubles and enactments, connected to the theme of summer, but I had to be spontaneous and work with what they were capable of doing. The purpose of the session was to show them what they *could* remember and to facilitate sharing wonderful memories.

Despite not having gone according to my original plan, the mission was accomplished. It was so simple and natural. We ended up with summer songs, juvenile jingles from Brooklyn, Philadelphia, London, Manchester and Australia. They were so happily surprised at how much they remembered in detail. Their associations succeeded in summoning up the colors, tastes, fragrances and the essence of summer into our room. They knew that they were remembering from the distant past to the recent past. Lila, feeling validated, proudly said, "I am defying the diagnosis. I do remember things. Thank you." She is no longer reticent. She trusts herself. She can speak up in our group.

> "I am defying the diagnosis.
> I do remember things. Thank you."

The Use of Metaphors

As I have mentioned, one criterion for picking a subject is the calendar. When we have a holiday, I help our participants connect to themselves, their past and their present via the significance of this ritualistic occasion.

The holiday after Chanukah is called Tu b'Shvat. It is the New Year for the trees; Israel's Arbor Day. What a great metaphor for exploring growth. The tree is often used as a metaphor to describe a person in Jewish culture. This is our theme for today's session. My goal is to raise awareness of what our participants do to grow and blossom.

I begin, "Yesterday we celebrated the holiday where we appreciate the trees that grow in Israel. In honor of this holiday, let's all enjoy transforming ourselves into the various trees all around our country." I use music from Tchaikovsky's Swan Lake that will help them express themselves through movement like a flourishing tree. I have discovered that this population enjoys escaping and distancing themselves from their reality.

When I ask them to make themselves as small as possible and then move the parts of their bodies to the rhythm of the music so that they can grow into trees, we are actually experiencing dance therapy adapted to this population. The music inspires the movement and they move their arms and torsos. We are all experiencing blossoming in nature through our bodies. We then meet the various trees and plants from all over the country and find out a bit about each one. We are in a safe aesthetic distance, ready to project. I use the metaphor and ask them to talk about themselves as the tree or plant they have become. This is also creative dramatics.

Just to give you an idea of how powerful this exercise can be, I will describe the most inspiring Creative Dramatics session in the course of my work with a group where dementia was not the issue. It took place during the Gulf War in 1991, and I was teaching creative dramatics to a group of women who were studying to get their teacher's degree. Scud missiles were falling around the country, and after two weeks of seeking the shelter of sealed rooms, wearing gas masks, the Ministry of Education decided to reopen the schools providing all students brought their personal gas masks with them and every school had a sealed room. Aside from their notebooks and tools for learning, each student carried a box that contained her personal gas mask – just in case there was a scud attack. I felt that I should find some therapeutic way to deal with the traumatic experience of war on the home front. I finally decided that I would do my session using trees as a metaphor in honor of *Tu b'Shvat*. In this session, I did a short guided imagery with the help of inspiring music to help the students transform into anything that grows in Israel and then tell us a piece of information – anything about themselves; where they are located, what fruit they bear, how they grow, what they look like.

I started the session as usual and after each tree told us their name, I said, "Wait . . . don't tell us about yourself. Please, tell us how you, as a tree, felt these past two weeks with scuds flying overhead."

What I was about to hear was astonishing. The trees that the young women portrayed covered every aspect of the Gulf War and provided deeply needed drama therapy for all us.

> "I am an apple tree, minding my own business on a street in Tel Aviv. (She stood with her arms straight above her head feeling light and empty.) All of a sudden, a strong swoosh went right through me and all my apples flew off. What was that!? I never felt anything so powerful and frightening before!"

> "I am on orange tree in an orchard in Rehovot. (She stood there hunched over with her arms portraying branches too heavy to bear.) Nobody is coming to pick my oranges. I can't support the weight. Where are the farmers?"

> "I am an almond tree. I am full of beautiful blossoms. I am so beautiful now. Every year at this time, kindergarten teachers bring little children to see me, to admire me, to photograph me. This year no one, but absolutely no one has come. Where are

all the children? Where are all the families? Where is everyone? What's going on? My blossoms will fall off shortly. No one is out. What a shame! I am so sad, so lonely. I look forward to these visits every winter."

"I am on old olive tree! (Her face is filled with dignity. Her arms are majestically outstretched.) My roots are thousands of years old. Nothing and no one will succeed to uproot me from here."

Coming back to our group of the elderly at Melabev, I use the metaphor as a tool for the deep, sensitive expression and interaction that they are capable of. I say to the participants, "Now that we have met all of these trees, let's think of why a tree would be sad." I become a sad tree for them saying, "I'm so very sad."

Lila–	Why are you so sad?
The sad tree:	"This used to be a beautiful forest but, some people were negligent and did not extinguish their picnic fires and the flames spread very quickly and all the beautiful trees around me are gone. Now I am all alone."
Monica–	God will help you.
Daisy–	A good rain.
Lila–	I'll plant you another tree so you won't be alone.
Daisy–	A tree is sad because it is growing old like an old person, not as useful as it used to be.
Lila–	I will hug you. Stay outside and get wet.
Daisy–	I don't think people get better as they get older. As you get older people respect you less.

This metaphor makes it easier for Daisy to express some deep emotions. The sad tree metaphor opens up a discussion of what makes *us* sad. The participants who don't usually express themselves and are happy to listen to the words of the other participants, suddenly find the courage to communicate freely and openly. What is more, they actually succeed, not without difficulty, to speak up. They know the other participants are interested in what they have to say. The metaphor of the tree develops into a discussion of what is deeply rooted in us and what we can replant and change in ourselves and in our lives. For example:

Daisy–	I'm working on not being a nuisance.
Lila–	I'm working on keeping busy and stimulating my mind.

Using the tree metaphor has been so valuable in enabling us to access and share buried emotions.

Reminiscence Therapy

Many of our sessions like Stories from Periods in Our Lives, Summertime, Winter, Imaginary Photo Album, The Use of Objects, and the Zoom session on the topic of Home, (See Table of Contents) were a form of Reminiscence Therapy which is often used to treat people with dementia. By reliving memories, the participants can reconnect, become engaged, are less withdrawn and feel more confident. Most of the memories were sentimental and heartwarming but we also encountered scenes that were filled with pain, regret, longing or anger. Through psychodrama, we were able to work them out. By using *surplus reality or future projection* our members were able to deal with unfinished business, guilt, shame and even trauma.

The Use of Objects

In one session, I bring my Chanukah Menorah. Over fifty years ago, my husband and I made this candelabra out of a piece of driftwood that we searched for and found in the Florida Keys. It is a precious item in our home because it was our work of art.

After sharing my personal story filled with the memories of this object, I ask the group, "Can you think of an item, an object, something in your home that is precious to you and which you cherish dearly?"

Here are a few of the precious objects which were mentioned:

Adrienne remembers her grandfather's bookcase filled with the Talmud and other Jewish scholarly works. Today, it is in the living room of her apartment.

Martin's son is a guest at this session and his father's eyes light up when he tells us about the candlesticks that his father gave him after his mother passed away about 12 years ago. He tells us that his wife lights the Sabbath candles with these silver candlesticks every Friday. Just hearing this makes Martin come alive. He is beaming. He shares his fond memories of these candlesticks which ushered in the Sabbath every week in his home throughout their marriage. This session took place nine months before Martin passed away. His health and cognition had declined severely. He would fall asleep during most of our sessions. Even in this session, with his son sitting next to him, he kept nodding off, but the moment his wife's silver candlesticks were mentioned he revived and remained awake until the end of this session.

Many of our participants connect to the word *silver* and we subsequently encounter other silver items.

Barbara has a lot of silver in her house. They are stored in a china closet.

Monica tells us that her grandfather gave her his grandfather clock that played music. She sings the song for the group and creates a magical moment for us.

Estelle, who has such a difficult time putting together a sentence, is so energized by these items that she is able to tell us a story with a sequence of sentences. Her paternal grandfather was a carpenter and he made breakfronts. A lot of his creations were shipped off before the war so that they would be saved. She gathers her thoughts and tells us that her grandfather survived the war and she has a lot of his carpentry in her home. She is reliving this victory, and we, in turn, are moved by her real victory in the ability to tell us this story.

Ruth tells us about a painting of her grandparents and their four children from Romania. It is on the bureau in her dining room. She tells us, very emotionally, that whenever she looks at it, she thinks of "the last good time together".

Geoffrey has a memory that tells us something about his early childhood.

> My mother and I escaped from Vienna and went to London before the war. My father didn't escape in time and did not survive the war. My father was a keen photographer and we had his camera. That made me feel connected to him. We also have a lot of letters between different people with communication about my father.

It is interesting that in the Zoom session about Home, he tells the story differently. He says that as a boy of two, he saw his father being shot and killed by the Nazis. For me, I am moved by the fact that he is capable of putting a sentence together and organizing what he is telling us.

Daisy connects to the pictures and to the silver candlesticks. She is a woman who is depressed and bitter because her family does not give her the nurturing she needs. She has a sentimental reminiscence triggered by the mention of a camera that brings a warm smile to her face as she shares it with us. She tells us that her father was a good photographer and he took a photo of her feeding her baby brother. This photo is hanging in her dining room. She adds that her grandmother gave her candlesticks. This sharing was a turning point for Daisy in our group. From hereon she participated actively and pleasantly in our sessions. She dressed more fashionably, with much more care and finesse. Her memory of being loved and showing love drew her out of her depressive state. Instead of sitting hunched over, her posture improved and she would sit up tall and proud. It was as if now, with her head held high, she can see the others in the group and is willing for the others to see her. She even started commenting on my attire and accessories. It was obvious that she was very intelligent and the group was an appreciative audience to her contributions. She felt nurtured and as a result was able to interact.

Deena is inspired and motivated from all the emotions in the room and the nostalgia. She talks about her son who passed away too young!

(See section on the telephone.) She has many photo albums of him and these are very precious to her.

Lionel tells us about Alfie, the family dog that his wife gave him after his dog, Freddie died. This dog actually showed up in another very memorable session in a role reversal where Lionel told us that his dog came to his daughter's wedding and, as a member of the family, was under the altar with all of them. Michal, our incredible volunteer, plays the dog. Through this role reversal, we learn what a faithful and significant friend this dog is to Lionel. The group loves the way Michal portrays the dog. Lionel relates to this portrayal as if the dog is truly talking to him and telling him of his devotion to Lionel.

Lionel is feeling very self-assured and empowered, thinking about his dog, and he points out that we keep on talking about things that people received when someone died. He asks us why we can't give things to our grandchildren while we are alive and we can see their enjoyment.

Simon shares that what is precious to him in his home is his wife. But he also cherishes the CDs of the famed singing rabbi, Rav Shlomo Carlebach that he has in his home.

Remembering objects shifts us from cherishing the past to appreciating the present. I never specifically asked for heirlooms but somehow most of the items were from their past. This session turned out to be *Reminiscence Therapy* and it definitely elicited elusive memories. Remembering, with the concrete image of items in their homes, brought out detailed descriptions with background stories. Some of the items that our participants remembered were so graphically described that we all felt we were in their homes with them. When a session evokes full participation and active listening, the participants gain a sense of belonging, vitality, value, power and intimacy. The staff was thrilled at this degree of expression.

Following is another session that illustrates the effective success of Reminiscence Therapy.

Remembering Special Moments in History

I open the session as follows, "We can write a history book based on events that occurred in our lives. Let's see what moments in history we can remember."

Lionel–	When I heard the words on the radio: "The Temple Mount is in our hands."
Pauline–	V-J day, August 15, 1945. We had just finished sitting shiva for my father. We were crossing a bridge but the traffic didn't move. There was an executive order to throw confetti.
Adrienne:	When I was 5 years old and England was at war.

Benjy: The Friday JFK was assassinated. The day Yitzhak Rabin was shot.

Barbara: The day Israel became a state, May 14, 1948.

Jennie: September 11, 2001.

Other responses mention the day John Lennon was killed, Princess Diana's death, when Meir Kahana was killed, Sputnik in the 1950s, when Natan Sharansky was freed, when the Soviet Union collapsed, when Neal Armstrong landed on the moon, 1989 and the fall of the Berlin wall. Who says we can't remember?!

This exercise was very empowering and enlightening. These recollections of events gave the participants a feeling of togetherness. They were being reminded of events they had all shared. Actually, this session was what Moreno called *Sociodrama* where the issues are collective and not personal. I could feel the group energy as different moments in history were remembered and shared. Everyone was involved and fully focused. As we opened up our discussion about these historical moments the participants were transported back to different periods in their lives.

I asked the participants to think of all of those days and continue remembering where they were and who was with them. We did a few short vignettes to bring us back to these moments. Our participants were energized and involved. The subject was so interesting and stimulating that they forgot about their disabilities and were feeling cognitively confident. Everyone participated.

Of course, by the next week, all of this was mostly forgotten. I never let that bother me. Each session with them was its own bloc of work. I would remind them of what was done before and help them connect but it did not necessarily register. When necessary I would weave the connecting thread so that it made sense to them at the moment. I would say, "Last week, or in the last few weeks, we worked on _____, now we will continue by working on _____." I would share my logic with them and they always approved and cooperated. As often as possible, I would remind people of what they had said or done in the previous session. Just hearing their names in this context is a form of validation.

Welcoming a New Member (an Account of Group Progress)

In this session, I learn how psychodrama has helped the participants develop their ability to communicate their truth and illustrate their innermost sensations. I have a very specific goal in this session. There is a new member in the group. He has early onset Alzheimer's disease. He is only 59. He attends the center for just two weekly sessions; a music session conducted by Howie, a very talented musician who was influential in his joining, and the Tuesday psychodrama session. I want him to see how helpful, dynamic, invigorating and entertaining our sessions can be. I am highly motivated to bring out the best in the group members, some of whom are 25 years older than him.

As I have sometimes done when new members join, I ask everyone in the group to introduce themselves to him and two other fairly new members and to add an adjective that describes their essence. This time, the adjectives are more substantial, precise and sophisticated. We have adjectives like cautious, inventive, ambitious and involved. Because it's now a higher level, some of the members are unable to find an apt description.

Here "trust the process" works. The other participants offer their suggestions and I also make my suggestions by doubling for them. Debra, the woman who complains a lot and can be nasty to the others (again, the names of the participants have been changed), sits there and simply says: "Oh I just don't know." My double for her is, "*I have so much pain and discomfort, and I'm frustrated.*" She agrees totally. This is an empathic experience for her. It is so true; she does not deny it. She owns it and it helps her, and the other group members understand her behavior. She actually has a smile on her face, a rare occurrence, as she restates, "Yes I am very frustrated." She receives validation. What a gift. It is also a gift to the group.

There is so much participation, involvement, sincere communication and interaction. And here is where the psychodrama proves its worth. For each trait, I ask the group to SHOW, with their hands, as if they have that trait on a scale from 1 to 10 and then indicate if they think they need that trait – from 1 to 10. This is a *sociometric spectrogram* without getting out of their seats. I then ask them to show, with their bodies and facial expression, how each trait is for them. They sculpt themselves and show the group what inventive, cautious, independent, etc. is for them. They are enacting. They are doing! They are internalizing, through action, in the comfort of their seats. And our new member is stimulated and *forgets* the age difference as he meets people who have so much in common with him and so much to share with him. Five years ago, this degree of engagement would not have seemed feasible for this "challenged" group of people.

Summary of Practical Applications

- Role reversals, small vignettes and doubles help our participants understand, internalize and release whatever is needed.
- Being open with the group is an invitation for the participants to also share. It is vital for the leader or facilitator in this group process, to not be distant or reticent.
- Sharing memories from the past stimulates identifying with one another via the world the participants grew up in.
- Objects from the home and events in history trigger expression and the sharing of special moments.

Part V

Understanding the Process

The Forms of Drama

Now that you have followed many sessions, and you know HOW they were conducted, I would like to explain, in my language and through concise quotes from the experts, the basic elements behind the various forms of drama. By *doing* in front of others, the participants gain self-confidence, a sense of belonging and an energy that helps overcome their limitations. This review should enable you to appreciate and apply drama in all its forms to your work.

As I stated in my introduction, I used creative dramatics, drama therapy and psychodrama in order to achieve the results you have just witnessed through the illustrations of our sessions. My main focus has been psychodrama but the other expressive art forms are woven in throughout our process. Without them, I would not have been able to be spontaneous in making adjustments to the special needs of our population. Whenever I have taught or given a workshop, I explain the basic differences between the forms of drama in order to avoid confusion and expand the options.

We will start from the beginning.

What Is Drama?

Whenever I start to work with a group, be it a course, workshop or therapy group, I want them to be prepared for the fact that in our sessions we will not be sitting back and listening. We will be active participants by *doing*. The groups can see my lineup of multicolored scarves on the tables behind me which is the first hint that something different is going to take place.

Just as I described in our opening session, I always open by saying, "First, what is drama? Drama is *doing*. The word drama is derived from the Greek *dram*, which means – a thing done."

I feel the response of the group. They are anticipating something new.

DOI: 10.4324/9781003321705-5

Here are some poignant quotes from world experts in these fields in order to give you, the readers, a deep sense and understanding of these techniques. These experts say it much better than me.

> From both an historical and developmental perspective, drama is a process of enactment that appears to be unlearned and indigenous to all human life.
>
> (Landy, 1994, p. 5)

> Drama is about extending boundaries of time and place as far as they can go and our emotional responses to them. It poses the question – what if? – allowing us to look at the possibilities of where a situation could lead if allowed to go to its limits, and alternative ways of getting there. The process is one of exploration through interaction and it happens in the present although we may be concerned with events of the past or the future.
>
> (Langley, 1994, p. 9).

Mc Niff compares drama to therapy. He states:

> Drama confronts and expounds upon human illusions, projected masks, false ideals, unconscious aggressions, suffering, death, loneliness, and all the emotional conflicts that surface in psychotherapy. Both therapy and drama are an affirmation of life, a "symbolic celebration" of human vitality through which the person *enacts* existential struggle while providing a structure in which struggle has meaning and value. True spontaneous drama created from the everyday lives of people is inherently therapeutic while psychotherapy is essentially a process of dramatic enactment.
>
> (Mc Niff, 1981, p. 207)

Elsewhere, he also says, "Dramatic enactment gives tangible form to a person's sense of being."

This is a general exposition. I will continue with the forms of drama.

Theater – All the World's a Stage

The origins of theater are in early religious rituals.

> Throughout the history of mankind there can be found traces of songs and dances in honor of a god, performed by priests and worshippers dressed in animal skins, and, of a portrayal of his birth, death, and resurrection. Theater, as we know it today, with a stage, an audience, and a rehearsed script delivered by actors to an audience in a special building or facility, was created by the Greeks in the fifth century BCE.

There are three elements necessary for theater as we know it today: (1) Actors who are performing (2) Conflict that is conveyed through dialogue (3) An audience emotionally involved in the action but not taking part in it.

(Hartnoll, 1985, p. 7)

The importance of emotional release is stressed by Landy:

> The ritual and healing aspects of theatre performance have been demonstrated throughout history. The theatre has been an institution for socially sanctioned emotional release, thought and debate, recreation, as people take a respite from everyday problems, and revolution, as people are propagandized or educated by participating in a particular dramatized point of view. . . . The theatre artist projects aspects of himself upon a fictional role which is then communicated to an audience.

(Landy, 1994, p. 49)

In modern theater, many of the norms have been challenged and altered, but the essential quality of actors performing to "entertain" an audience has remained. This book deals with relationships and activities in the environment of a daycare center for senior citizens coping with many debilitating challenges. Dorothy Heathcote, a pioneer in drama in education, pointed out the difference between drama and theater for classroom purposes: "The difference between theater (performance) and classroom drama is that in theater everything is contrived so that the audience gets the *kick*" (Wagner, 1976, p. 147). In our sessions, the participants got the *kicks*. These *kicks* are the results of what I have been describing. I never use the words to act or to perform. I always say "show us". In many ways, our room is a classroom. We even have a blackboard and a bookcase. There is a bulletin board on which their activity schedule for the week is written, much like in a classroom environment.

The benefits of using theater with groups, where there is a stage, a text and an audience, are varied. The actors get to identify with the characters they are portraying and with the conflicts in the plot. They are exposed to stimulating stories and intrigues. They experience group work, cooperation, language development, catharsis and creativity and achieve satisfaction through working towards a common goal. If we would want to create a theater performance with our group, it would be impossible for obvious reasons. The participants in this group are not capable of remembering texts or even reading the words of their roles in a play. Not to mention the physical obstacles in staging a scene. We can however expose them to good theater and let them see a play together and follow up with many invigorating discussions and activities. Also, the technical aspects of developing a theatre performance with a director, producer, actors, scenery, props and costumes is a project that is financially and practically inadvisable. We do, however, have other options. One of them is discussed in the following section.

Creative Dramatics

Before I became a psychodramatist, my field was Creative Dramatics. But more of that a little later in this section. Whether in an educational or recreational framework, creative dramatics has as its goals: awareness of ourselves, one another, and our environment through creative activities such as games, exercises, and improvisations. The creative *process*, rather than the product, is the goal. It can be therapeutic but healing is not a goal. It can be aesthetic, entertaining and memorable but the end product is a side effect and not a goal. It is not a performance. There should be no audience. It is a socializing activity where one spontaneously discovers and interacts. Brian Way calls it a "system of training in life skills" (Bolton, 1984, p. 59) According to Cottrell, the basis for creative dramatics is the use of imagination. She maintains:

> To become someone or something else requires the player to imagine how another thinks, feels, moves, communicates, values, and relates to others and to the world. Children involved in drama use their minds to image objects and events not present to their senses. They become creative thinkers who are able to invent solutions to problems through the synthesizing of new ideas from perceptions previously experienced separately and to express those ideas through the drama. Creative dramatics is a group art that encourages children to share the offerings of their imaginations through social interaction. For if intelligence without imagination is useless, we might also add that intelligence without communication is a waste of the greatest magnitude. Communication is, of course, our greatest source of knowledge of self and of others and is basic to social order.
>
> (Cottrell, 1987, Introduction)

In this quote, we can see that we can achieve many of the goals of performing in a play without the tension, fuss, expense and difficulty of a theater stage. Even though the reference here is to children, drama therapy works successfully with our population. Remember, I stated that my original plan was to make this book one chapter in a book called *Drama With Mama: A Handbook on How to Use Drama With Children of All Ages*.

Before studying psychodrama, I studied Drama in Education in a Master's program at N.Y.U. The bibliography of this book is filled with references that apply to drama in the classroom. Much of this was very applicable and successful with this population. When I taught student teachers and teachers getting their Master's degrees, I discovered that adults also need, enjoy and thrive on creative dramatics.

Moreover, when I studied drama therapy and psychodrama, I discovered how therapeutic creative drama was. I used creative drama with children and adults for over 30 years and incorporated it into my new profession. It has definitely been woven into many of our sessions. All those years of working with hundreds of children, kindergarten through high school, teachers and students studying for these professions, gave me a vast repertoire of exercises, games, techniques, resourcefulness, exposure to all kinds of populations, and experience which came in very handy in this new stage of my career.

As we move on, we must note the difference between drama therapy and psychodrama. First, look at the two terms. *Drama* therapy emphasizes the word drama, while *Psycho*drama emphasizes the word psycho. These two forms of expressive therapy often overlap but each therapeutic technique has its unique method and goal.

Drama Therapy

It is difficult to define drama therapy, because of "the emphasis on spontaneity, creativity, and play, which, by necessity, leaves a lot of freedom for experimentation and change" (Kedem-Tahar and Kellerman, 1996, p. 28). Although experts in this field like Jennings, Landy, Emunah, Chesner and Langley have tried to systemize and find definitions, there is no general agreement. In pointing out the basic philosophical differences between psychodrama and drama therapy, Kedem-Tahar and Kellerman actually give an apt distinction: "Whereas in psychodrama the *soul* (psyche) is the aim and the *action* (drama) *is* the means, the opposite is true for dramatherapy in which drama itself (as pure art) is the aim and the psyche is the means of expression" (ibid. p. 29). They claim:

> Most practitioners probably agree that drama therapy refers to the utilization of dramatic methods in group situations, usually for the general purposes of promoting *healing* intrinsic to art, developing skills of improvisation and creative thinking, expanding the repertoire of roles with the inclusion of body movement and other aesthetic dimensions. From a technical point of view, drama therapists use a wide range of exercises built on music, movement, sound, mime, physical relaxation, narratives, guided daydreaming, imagery and play. Often, various stage props such as dolls, masks, costumes, make-up and inanimate objects, are used as imaginary stimulation for dramatization of stories and myths, detailed improvisation of situations or the enactment and exploration of classical texts.
>
> (ibid. pp. 28–29)

And here are some additional quotes from experts in drama therapy which can strengthen and underscore all that I have shown in this book.

In discussing what healing is in drama therapy, Emunah states:

> Given the complexity and challenge of living, we cannot afford to exist without a highly developed sense of *empathy* and perspective. We need to understand not only ourselves but the motivations, drives and feelings of the *other* players in our lives – in order to improve our interactions, relationships, and social structures. I know no better way to understand the experience of another than by putting myself *in his or her shoes*. Becoming another person through dramatic enactment is much more powerful and effective than imagining in my mind that person's situation. Drama, by its very nature, induces empathy and perspective.
>
> (Emunah, 1994, p. xv)

And she goes on to say, "Drama therapy invites us to uncover and integrate dormant aspects of ourselves, to stretch our conception of who we are, and to experience our intrinsic connection with others" (ibid., p. xvii).

Drama, as therapy, can produce change and healing through creativity. According to Langley (1983), drama helps promote growth, change, and healing through trust, group cohesion, memory, role-play, learning social skills, relaxation, sensory perception and physical awareness, concentration and communication. McNiff tells us:

> Through drama we move and express conflict, we transform our struggles into a form which is conveyed to ourselves and to other people, and we experience the total catharsis and release that can be obtained only through the *enactment*, which draws upon the full expressive powers of the organism.
>
> (Mc Niff, 1981, p. 209)

Just like youngsters, the people in our group loved playing roles that were not possible in the reality of their daily lives, such as gangsters, seductive sexy ladies, business tycoons, rebellious teenagers, athletic stars. Whenever we improvised situations with fictional characters, there was a lightness in the room and an atmosphere of fun. They enjoyed escaping their limited lives and pretending in our improvisations. More than the frolic, this was therapeutic for them. Robert Landy wrote a book: *Persona and Performance: The Meaning of Role in Drama, Therapy and Everyday Life* (1993), where he gives fascinating clinical illustrations and theoretical explanations of the value of playing an array of roles through drama therapy sessions. These sessions, with our group, were difficult to document because the rhythm of the action and the language of the participants was too quick to record. Our writers were enjoying spontaneity. They were watching instead of writing. The indelible impression left from these drama therapy sessions was of a total release and letting go through vicarious made-up situations. Everything that you just read in the above quotes was definitely realized whenever I would come in to the room and announce, "Today, we are going to pretend."

One of the subtle but significant benefits of using drama with the elderly has to do with the new role in their life. A person suffering from senile dementia sees himself as not normal, incapable, dependent even irrational. This self-image has become their new role in life. Whereas this person lived a normative life, built a family, had a successful career, was involved in a social community and contributed to society, today he sees himself as unfit. This too is a new role. Through drama in all its forms, this person discovers roles other than the elder, the demented or the incapable. Yes, he is an older adult but with a better self-image.

In these sessions, we have witnessed their new sense of being meaningful. They experience validation when the group acts as a mirror as they see one another performing and functioning. They learn self-esteem as they enact various roles in dramatic settings together; they receive options. They are empowered by *doing*. Sometimes simply announcing who they would like to be has this effect on them. They become aware of their potential despite their limitations. They enjoy their new roles in our sessions because for 75 minutes they can discard the role of the incapable old man or woman and be . . . anything and anyone. Robert Landy shows the possibility for growth through role exploration via drama throughout his book. Under the circumstances, we can't really have a continuum with people who can't remember. Despite this, the participants gain a new self-image through identification with the other members and through experiencing new roles.

To watch the participants move out of the role of the fragile, forgetful, dependent, useless old person into the role of the powerful lawyer, doctor, leader, scoundrel, aide, son, granddaughter or an imaginary role of dancer, tennis star or a baby, is to watch an outpouring of pure joy. There were many instances where there was even a glimmer of integration between the roles played in our sessions and their difficult reality.

Psychodrama

Psychodrama is a form of psychotherapy developed by J. L. Moreno in the 1920s. Moreno was impressed with the way children were able to act out stories and express deep emotions in activity groups. (He, too, was inspired through children.) He demonstrated that "by enacting ideas and situations an individual can understand them more deeply and can gain insight into his own feelings" (Stanford and Roark, 1974, p. 171). He saw the "oneness of theater and therapy . . . as an artistic enactment of the living process" (Mc Niff, 1981, p. 217). He developed a form of psychoanalytical psychotherapy by first forming a "theater of spontaneity". He called this technique psychodrama and defined it as "an exploration of truth through dramatic methods" (Langley, 1983, p. 19).

According to Kellerman:

> Psychodrama is a method of psychotherapy in which clients are encouraged to continue and complete their actions through dramatization, role playing, and dramatic self-presentation. Both verbal and non-verbal communications are utilized. A number of scenes are enacted, depicting, for example, memories of specific happenings in the past, unfinished situations, inner dramas, fantasies, dreams, preparations for future risk-taking situations, or unrehearsed expressions of mental states in the here and now. These scenes either approximate real-life situations or are externalizations of inner mental processes. If required, other roles may be taken by group members or by inanimate objects. Many techniques are employed such as role reversal, doubling, mirroring, concretizing, maximizing and soliloquy. Usually the phases of warm-up, action, working through, closure and sharing can be identified.
>
> (Kellerman, 1992, p. 20)

A Classical Psychodrama Session

Even though psychodrama played a major role in my work with this group, I could never use psychodrama in its full classical form in my work at Melabev. Many psychodramatists around the world are guided by what is called "The Hollander Curve" which was developed by Carl Hollander (1937–2003). This is a model that is meant to be dynamic and used as a general outline for a full group session. A full psychodrama with a group requires two to three hours. These sessions are very powerful. I will briefly describe what happens in a classical group psychodrama session according to the Hollander Curve. We start with a warm-up. The warm-up in classical psychodrama induces spontaneity in order to generate creativity and produce a theme. Hopefully, a protagonist emerges. There are many methods to choose the protagonist. Sometimes the director will ask the group directly: Who wants or needs to "work" today? My psychodrama groups knew that everyone will have a chance to declare what they need to work on. Sometimes it is obvious to everyone who will be the protagonist. Other times, the group chooses the protagonist according to how much the subject raised will also work for them. Sometimes I know that a particular person must work today on something that is causing deep distress. The group always agrees to let that person "work".

We then interview the protagonist and after understanding the conflict, dilemma, cause of distress or issue, we bring it to action. We call this the *enactment*. In this phase of the Hollander Curve, we have a first scene where we explore and expose the reality. We create a setting for the scene: first, we establish the time; season, date and hour. We then let the protagonist describe the place and physically set it up by providing a few details about the place with some tangible props so that the protagonist can deeply connect to the setting and *be there*. For example, if it is in the backyard of the home, I will ask, "What do you see in your backyard? What furniture is there in your backyard? Where is the barbeque? Where do you sit?" We just need a few symbolic props to help the protagonist become emotionally connected to the setting. We then bring the people into the scene. The protagonist does the casting. This is the protagonist's warm-up. This first scene exposes and explores the problem.

We then develop a second scene in the same way. It is usually a scene from the past where the protagonist might reach an emotional peak or a catharsis or at least an action insight.

We then have a third scene where we aim for closure. We might return to the setting in the first scene or use surplus reality and make up a situation that will help the protagonist reach a positive ending to this exposing enactment.

We then move on to the third stage, which is called "integration". This is where we have the group share how they connected to this entire psychodrama. The sharing has two purposes. Firstly, the enactment they just witnessed and even might have participated in may trigger associations with the protagonist's experience. They can then tell the protagonist and the group their *story*. I have an acquaintance who lost a child tragically. Her therapist recommended that she join a psychodrama grief group. She told me that there was no way she would ever be a protagonist but the sharing helped her talk about her grief and post-trauma issues. She felt safer with this.

The second reason for sharing is to help the protagonist learn that other group members also have issues that need to be addressed. The protagonist will feel less exposed and vulnerable through this sharing.

With this group, it would have been impossible to "hold" them in such a dynamic session. I am briefly describing it so that you can understand the background to how I conducted our sessions using some of these stages and techniques, whenever possible, in order to help our group members reach new insights through action and connect to themselves and one another through these enactments that I have documented for you.

In all these years with this group, I used the tools of psychodrama: *role reversals, doubles, vignettes, enactments, sharing, sociometry, spectrograms, surplus reality* and combined them with the techniques of drama therapy in order to facilitate *doing* instead of simply talking about different subjects. Just the fact that these participants followed some of the rules of psychodrama, like allowing a role reversal, listening to their doubles, or waiting till the end of the enactment to share, was a major accomplishment.

Moreno's language was very familiar to all of them: "trust the process", "don't tell me, show me", "theater of truth". These were phrases that they all adopted and shared throughout our activities.

Even though psychodrama, is very powerful, I used its techniques and tools in a way that was safe and appropriate for our group. It was necessary for the staff and the volunteers to participate. We used humor and playfulness in our psychodrama enactments but, the fact that the material was from their actual lives made these sessions more direct and more serious in nature.

Summary of Practical Applications

- Familiarizing yourself with the various forms of drama, and their application to this population will equip you with more exercises and methods of working with the elderly and with people suffering from dementia.
- Creative Dramatics, Drama Therapy and Psychodrama can be interlaced into a typical session in order to contribute to the therapeutic quality of the action and interaction.
- Drama, in all its forms, by its very nature, can generate understanding, empathy and deep insights.

Understanding Heinz Kohut

As you already know, I *do*! I am a very active creature. The doctors and psychologists who have attended our sessions attest to the fact that all this *doing* and interaction is very beneficial emotionally and medically to our participants. They were sure that there is a way to measure this progress, but this book is a handbook – a guide on what we can *do* to improve social cohesion and self-efficacy. For readers who are not familiar with Heinz Kohut's technical terms, used in this book, I will try to explain them in the following section, in a way that can be better understood and utilize this information beneficially.

The psychological basis for almost all of my work is Kohut's self-theory. After reading and learning about his innovative approach to the development of a healthy self-image, I was able to adapt the essence of his work to my work in classrooms, psychodrama groups and my clinical practice.

For me, what is essential is his understanding that a healthy self is the result of basic factors in the natural intuitive relationship between a mother or caretaker and an infant. I originally was planning to write a book called *Drama with Mama*, a handbook on how drama, in all its forms, can help the development of children of all ages, through techniques and exercises that bring about *empathy, twinship, mirroring and grandiosity*. This approach has been the backbone of the goals in my work.

This is how I understand Kohut's contribution to a healthy development of the self that can be applied to using drama in a therapeutic manner. I am repeating it here because it is so essential to my philosophy: everyone needs to experience *empathy, twinship, mirroring and grandiosity*. These basic concepts are inherent in the mother-infant relationship. If a person's basic needs are not met, it will affect the way he relates to himself and to others in the future. These concepts can be used as genuine tools of communication and connection anywhere that people are interested in enhancing the lives of others.

I will now explain each concept in the context of my work.

Empathy

Empathy is the capacity to think and feel oneself into the inner life of another person. It is our lifelong ability to experience what another person experiences (Kohut, 1984, p. 82). It is the ability of the therapist to see the world from the client's point of view. Although it usually comes naturally to a mother in her relationship to her baby, it is not necessarily intuitive and a person's capacity for empathy can grow through training and learning. A mother can use her empathy to know and respond to her children. An actor will spend hours of training so that he can get a deeper experience of how the character he is portraying might think or feel in different situations. In this way, his acting is more than a mere imitation. A director will guide his actors through an empathic understanding of what the actor is experiencing as he is deeply immersed in the portrayal of his character. Similarly, a teacher can be made aware of the learning needs of a pupil and a therapy group director can feel the immediate needs of participants.

Empathy is not how we might feel if we were in the same situation. It is the experience of putting ourselves in the inner world of others in order to truly understand and communicate effectively. It is being someone who understands someone else's feelings. It is much deeper than being nice and appearing sympathetic. Empathy acknowledges the existence of the other. It affirms their humanness. In the caretaker–child relationship, it is expressed in the caretaker's touching and smelling while holding the child close, and progresses to a more distant holding through words and facial expression. I always give my students the example of my daughter and her first baby (my first grandchild, who was born in 1998). When the baby was three months old, I offered to babysit so that my daughter and her husband could have an evening out, and go see a show at the theater near our home. My daughter had full trust that I would babysit with no problem. About an hour after she left, the baby woke up and started screaming. I tried everything to calm her down. Nothing worked. I checked her diaper, tried a pacifier and offered a bottle. The screaming got louder and would not stop. I danced. I pranced.

I rocked. Nothing worked. This was in 1998, many years ago. There were no cellphones in our family but the home phone rang. It was NOT the intermission of the show. My daughter had walked out of the theater, in the middle of the first act. She went to the public phone in the lobby (remember them??). She asked: "Is she crying?" I was sure she could hear the baby's screaming from the theater which was a mere ten-minute walk from our home! I answered: "How did you know?" Her answer was, "I could feel it. My baby needs me. I could not enjoy the play. I am coming back." This was *empathy*. The mother felt her baby's need for her. It was built in. And I could feel her distress – which spoke to my empathy as her mother! I was stunned by this event.

Empathy in Our Group

I read somewhere that the genuineness of empathy involves trust over criticism and hope over judgment. By feeling truly understood and understandable, the participant is encouraged to develop his capabilities. By feeling accepted and worthwhile, the person is encouraged to devote himself wholeheartedly to his own advancement, despite the daily, ever-increasing challenges. Affording an empathic environment between the people in our circle also builds a sensitivity to everyone's individual fundamental needs.

The best example of empathy in our circle was the *double* where I would physically stand behind the person after they said something. I would first ask, "Would you like a *double* here?" No one ever said no. They loved to hear a double on whatever it was they said. The double said what I perceived that person was feeling but not saying. This tool was very applicable in this group because so many of the participants had difficulty in retrieving the words that could express what they were trying so hard to say. The double found the words for them. Sometimes the double elaborated more deeply. Other times a few words were enough to let them know I understood empathically what they were feeling and helped them share this feeling with the group. I have brought many examples in descriptions of our sessions. Here's one: Deena was also suffering from paranoia, on top of her dementia. Every time I would turn to her for her response, she would blush crimson. Her body would shrink inwards as much as physically possible and she would respond, in a self-conscious whisper, with the untranslatable Yiddish expression – *oy vey*. The closest translation would be 'woe is me.' This *oy vey* received my *double* reframing her thoughts, "*Oh I don't know what to say, No one believes me. I am too old to express myself. I don't want to say something stupid. Maybe I didn't understand your direction.*"

Her response affirmed how true this was for her.

Often the double said what the participants would not venture to say and helped them release deep feelings of frustration or need. The double could also help them reach new insights into their situations. One of my goals was to let them do doubles for one another. I am not giving up on this goal. Many times, I ask "Would any of you like to try and do a double for_____?" So far, only the staff and volunteers have responded, albeit infrequently, but I have faith that it could happen. In my other groups, it is common practice. But this group was very different from all my other psychodrama groups. Even with my other groups, though, it took time before people would find the courage and know-how to do doubles.

Role reversal develops empathy with the person they are portraying. When Barbara role-reversed and played her aide, she understood that her aide wants to help her but needs time to get to know her needs.

All of our *sharing*, after every psychodramatic *enactment*, led to empathy. Sharing, in psychodrama, is a method where everyone tells (shares) how they connected with what they just witnessed so that the protagonist is not the only one feeling exposed. Empathy is, indeed, a major element in our sessions and fills a deep need in this population.

Mirroring

A child feels special, wonderful, loved, wanted and welcome when his parents give him *mirroring* through a subtle gesture, expression or a tone of voice. It is when the child is looked at by the mother and he looks at her. The gleam in the mother's eye is a response to the child's actions and sends a message of approval. Today, unfortunately, children are starved of this vital mirroring, so necessary to the next stage of their development. Their needs are competing with cellphones and all the modern screens: iPhones, computers, iPads, television sets, etc.

In healthy development, the grandiose exhibitionist behavior of the child is encouraged by the mother's mirroring and is a confirmation of the child's self-esteem. It feeds into the narcissistic exhibitionism of the child as a natural, healthy stage of development. This is where Kohut's "legitimizing" of narcissism begins. This theory applies beautifully to our group and its inherent needs.

> Mirroring is a glance, a touch and attention. It can also be auditory where the sound echoes just as a mirror reflects. We learn from this that 'the analyst' (in this case, the psycho-dramatist) is the well-delimited target of the patient's demands that he will reflect, echo, approve, and admire his exhibitionism and greatness.
>
> (Kohut, 1971, p. 147)

Everyone needs mirroring, and in the therapist–client relationship, it is essential according to self-psychology. I have seen that all of this applies to the people I am working with at Melabev and is implemented in our group sessions of psychodrama therapy.

I would always demonstrate the mirroring of a mother and a baby to my students by asking them to show us how we feed a baby in a high chair. We take the spoon and move it towards the baby's mouth and we open our mouth instinctively as the baby opens its mouth to receive the portion of food. It is incredible and foolproof. It happened every time I did this. Everyone opened their mouth!

Mirroring in our circle is a verbal or nonverbal gesture, message, cue or response that evokes a sense of approval. It gives the feeling that someone is *with* you. It affords reassurance through a subtle glance or movement or sound. It is undefined encouragement and indirect affirmation. It is not an evaluation but, rather, a reflection, and a confirming and validating response. Mirroring can occur, rather easily, between the participants and the group leader (in this case – me, but hopefully, after you read this – you). There are many opportunities to be spontaneous and flexible and to acknowledge and recognize specifically what the participant is communicating. She or he receives a positive message of approval and appreciation through simple mirroring when a person's accomplishment is repeated, or when artwork is displayed on a bulletin board. Likewise, a nod of the head, a facial expression, a leaning forward or an opening of arms towards the participant sends a message of yes, Yes, YES! In order to achieve mirroring between group members, it is necessary to apply specific techniques from something as basic as altering the seating arrangement, to providing numerous opportunities for them to see and hear each other within the environment of our circle. Sitting in a circle and seeing everyone affords many opportunities for them to experience mirroring so that they, too, can acknowledge and affirm what is being said and done by the others in the group.

When someone repeats a person's action, word, movement or sound, that person will experience mirroring. In our population, where so many have hearing problems, it is interesting to see how a person responds to, "What did she say? I want to hear. Please repeat it." The person, who was not heard clearly, sits taller and repeats what was said much louder and clearer, with a sense of importance. I am not sure this is what Kohut meant but, through this interaction, they are definitely experiencing mirroring.

Mirroring Exercises

Many of the drama exercises are actually mirroring games that require people to observe each other carefully, and repeat one another's movements and echo each other's sounds.

Here are some more examples of mirroring through exercises. Firstly, a mirroring basic arrangement of the space – the circle – enables imitation in group work.

Mirroring and holding occur when each person looks at everyone in the circle. Sometimes, I ask all of the participants and the staff to hold hands and establish eye contact with every other person in the circle. This sounds simple but, believe me, it is challenging.

All of the name games that we do, afford mirroring, such as the game where we throw a pillow to someone after describing something about them (see the section in PART II Following Session: Developing Cohesion in the Group).

Saying your name and adding an action that depicts something you like to do. The next person repeats what you did and then continues. With this group, I need to be one second ahead of them for it to proceed successfully, but they are definitely exercising their memory cells through mirroring! Throughout the book, in the elaboration of sessions, I have mentioned this therapeutic occurrence.

Each person says his name and pantomimes an activity he recently enjoyed doing or something that he likes or dislikes doing or something he did over the weekend, summer, etc. or something that is easy to do, with a movement. The person to his right will repeat his name and mirror what he just did and add his name and his movement.

After each person has presented his name plus a movement, we start stage two of this group mirroring exercise. One person in the group repeats one of the movements, without looking at the originator of this movement. The other participants join in by continuously mirroring the movement together. When ALL of them have mirrored the original movement, the originator proceeds by moving on and mirroring someone else's movement. This continues until all of the movements have been mirrored. Each person experiences a mirroring of a personal expression of his likes and dislikes etc., as displayed in his pantomime. Also, mirroring occurs when each person experiences the entire group imitating *his* movement and looking at *him*.

Another mirroring game is Name Statues:

a. Participant #1 says his name and freezes in a position that he chooses.
b. Participant #2 precisely copies #1's position, repeats #1's name and then adds his name and his own position.
c. Participant #3 copies #1 and #2 and adds her name and her own position. After three, the first person sits down, so that no one has to mirror more than three people and that is truly demanding. Each person experiences a mirroring of his personal statue and hears his name echoed two or three times by other members of his group which is a visual and an audio form of mirroring.

In the Hat of Fear exercise (see that section), when we hear what was written in the notes that were placed in the hat, we experience *audio* mirroring.

Seeing everyone responding to what one has just said is itself a form of mirroring. Every time the participants raise their hands from 0 to 10 when I ask who else feels this way. Show us by where your hand is from 0 to 10.

When someone remembers a song from long ago and starts singing and everyone joins in for the chorus, as happened many times, in our sessions, we get another form of mirroring.

When the group works in pairs and I invite them to share something between them and then I instruct them to tell us what they learned from their partner, we have another form of mirroring. Each person and the entire group hear what was shared with the partner. Obviously, all the effects of connecting and feeling less socially isolated are results of these subtle, but fun, forms of mirroring.

The most natural mirroring exercise is where two people stand or sit opposite each other and do simple movements together as if one is the mirror of the other. At some point, they switch and the second person becomes the mirror. I start by doing the mirror exercise with one person in order to demonstrate. That person, A., will mirror my simple flowing movements. This already will be an accomplishment. I then ask A. to be the leader and I follow A.'s movements as if I am that person's mirror. I then ask two volunteers to do the same exercise with two or three other people in the group. If I see that they are enjoying the mirroring connection, I then divide them into pairs where the staff and I partner with the people who are challenged and the rest of the group does it on their own. If this works, I further challenge them by announcing "switch" a few times until they are capable of continuing without knowing who the leader is and who is the mirror. This kind of exercise also creates an exciting *twinship*.

Twinship

Whenever we divide the group into pairs or small groups, they can experience *twinship*. They achieve a sense of belonging and, more important, a sense of alikeness, sameness and bonding that are difficult to achieve in their deteriorating situation. To achieve this sense of "we are alike", or "I am not alone", it is necessary to let the participants work together on drama exercises – large or small, minor or major – to create social cohesion.

To achieve this sense of "We are alike", or "I am not alone", it is necessary to let the participants work together on exercises – large or small, minor or major – to create social cohesion.

All the exercises that we have been doing help achieve this essential feeling of "us". The exercises carried out in pairs and in small groups of four form the bond called *twinship*. So just as work in pairs, where the person tells the group what the partner revealed, enabled audio mirroring, the simple task of sharing about a subject enabled *twinship*. There were also occasions where the subject was about the handling of an uncomfortable dilemma and how we address such situations in our daily lives. The bond that is created in partner work makes it easier to open up comfortably and divulge to the partner and then share with the group. Working in pairs was ideal for newer members who still needed intimacy with one person plus time with the group to build trust.

Just think of this word **twin** . . . ship. Twins usually are remarkably aligned and in touch with the feelings of one another. That is the goal of these exercises. Kohut showed how, with the help of empathy and mirroring, he was able to establish a bond of *twinship* with his patients. A mother or caretaker gives the baby a sense of belonging. As the child grows, family rituals give the child the security of knowing what will happen at specific hours and on specific days or occasions. A few of our routines and rituals in our sessions helped the participants feel like a family. My Group knew that on Tuesday mornings at 10:15 something very bonding was going to happen. They were aware that now they would be doing something together. They would be sharing and showing. They had achieved a deep and secure sense of belonging. This is probably why they loved these sessions. *Twinship* is the remedy for loneliness, and it works for every age.

Sharing – From My Process With Adolescents

A sweet anecdote here might help explicate *twin* . . . *ship*. I would often exclaim to my students that twins are especially attuned to one another. If I would ask two students to come forward, close their eyes, and when they feel it is the right time, to raise their right hand, it usually will not be together. If I would ask twins to do this, especially identical ones – they would probably succeed in doing this together. A few times, I was challenged by the fact that there were twins in that particular group that I was teaching. Each time this happened I had no choice but to do this experiment right there and then. Each time, everyone was pleasantly surprised to see the twins move together in exactly the same rhythm. Yes, this is *twinship* at its zenith.

With our group, I would sometimes ask them to close their eyes and try to feel when would be the right time to clap their hands together. It was a challenge that created its own form of twinship.

There is a simple game that this group loved. I was surprised at the level of participation. I clap my hands and someone says the number 1. Then someone else says the number 2 followed by the number 3 and so on. But, if two people say a number together, we start all over from the beginning. Surprisingly, even the most passive members of the group participated and tried their luck. All they have to do in order to be a part of this experience is to say a number. They were very alert and connected and we actually succeeded in reaching the number 10. Some of their mistakes were caused by innate confusion but an atmosphere of laughter and frolic was created by the slips.

In order to better understand how this game works, and encourage you to try it with your families, I would like to present an experience with three different classes of thirty girls. This game is very applicable and informative for all groups. Whenever I used this game, in a classroom, I would then give the class a free diagnosis whereby they could learn about themselves. In my work with these three seventh-grade classes, as an introduction to my meetings with them, I would start out by telling the girls that in our sessions there is no book, no blackboard, and no notebook. They are the book and their homework would be to think of what they learned about themselves, about one another and about the group as a whole from our psychodrama sessions. I told them that one of the aims of our sessions is to turn them into a jazz ensemble. I would ask, "What is the difference between an orchestra and a jazz ensemble?" After many attempts to find the difference, such as different types of music, or number of players, I would explain:

> In an orchestra there is a conductor and there are notes. You girls sit in this classroom facing the blackboard and the teacher conducts you in order to produce your beautiful music with intricate arrangements – like an orchestra! She needs texts and you need her directing. In a jazz ensemble, there's no conductor and no written music. The musicians feel the rhythm, the beat. They create the harmony by connecting, by feeling when is it me, when is it she? When is it fast, slow? When is it together, solo, duet? They are so attuned, that they know when and how. The music is dynamic. The experience is exciting, vitalizing and fulfilling. That's what I want to happen here, in your classroom. You won't raise your hand here. You will know when to speak and when to listen. It will be so relaxing and reassuring and nice to be together with so many girls and to know that you will have a place, a voice, a presence and you will enjoy what others have to contribute to the class concert.

The seventh-grade girls understood because I believed in what I was telling them. So, the process of becoming a "jazz ensemble" and experiencing a form of twinship had begun. In order to check how much work each of these three groups needed in order to function together like a "jazz ensemble", we played this same simple but informative counting game. Here is a more elaborate description of the process to make sure you can do this.

I say:

> We are going to count, all of us, 1, 2, 3 etc. But if more than one girl says a number, we start over from 1. Here goes. I will clap my hands and then one of you will say the number 1 and another will say 2. We will aim to get to at least 10. There were groups that couldn't get to the number 2.

> Clap.
> "One"
> Clap.
> "Two"
> Clap.
> "Three" "Three"
> Whoops – start all over again.

I ask the students – "Who said the number 1 more than once?" Usually, two to three of them raise their hands. I also ask who said any number more than three to four times and again usually, a small number of students raise their hands. I then give two options for diagnosis and they can figure out for themselves which diagnosis is appropriate for whom, without singling out any individual.

> Perhaps you are an initiator, a leader, you want action, you are not afraid of ruining things for the group, you like the whole idea of playing games or it simply helps you feel involved. On the other hand, you could be interested only in yourself; I want, I need, center stage. I don't see or care about anyone else. Maybe it's all about me Me ME! The rest of you be quiet.

I see subtle smiles on some faces as they understand and internalize the message.

I then ask who did not even say one number. I give them two options for a diagnosis. I tell them that either they are very thoughtful and magnanimous and they want the group to succeed so, if they keep quiet, there is a better chance of that happening, or, on the other hand, perhaps they are saying to themselves that they are not taking a chance. They are afraid of ruining this for the class. They are protecting themselves. Everyone knows who this applies to. What they all internalize is important information.

This gives us a pretty clear picture of the situation in the classroom. Often, an overwhelmingly large number of students raise their hands. I then know what kind of work is cut out for me with this group, to strengthen the passive students and help make room for them in this group.

This diagnosis describes four personalities that exist in almost every typical classroom in various versions. I say, "So, which one are you? Check if you are any of these personalities and think of what you can do to be more balanced in your interactions." By their attention and the look in their eyes, I know they have heard me.

The diagnosis here also helped exemplify different aspects of our participants' personalities that are not written in their files. We had a diagnosis through observing their behavior in this game. I presented the information more tactfully or not at all. It helped to serve as a diagnostic tool for the staff. There were a few who kept on saying the numbers 1 and 2, with gusto and assurance. Surprisingly, everyone got to say a number. Everyone took an active part in this activity. If you try this with your family, you will thank me. And yes, our group functioned like a "jazz ensemble".

Grandiosity

Grandiosity for Kohut is quite different from our usual perception of this word. For Kohut, grandiosity is when the participant in a group is given the "floor" and the leader encourages him to enlarge and "go with it" – become a star! That person is urged to dare. This is his legitimate opportunity for more and more. Grandiosity requires an audience. Drama in the group is a very suitable vehicle for the expansion, enlargement and enhancement of the individual's performance in front of the group. He will achieve a sense of pride and achievement through the direct or indirect applause of the others. He will have witnesses who will satisfy his exhibitionistic need. So, forget about your preconception of the word grandiosity as pompous and imposing. In this context, we will go with Kohut and see how grandiosity helps build confidence through applause.

When a baby takes its first step, what happens? Everyone gets excited and cheers the baby on. The baby feels this positive energy and tries another step. Very soon, a penguin is born! With head held high, the baby is ready to lunge ahead. This is true of children of all ages. Our participants LOVED being in the limelight – the essence of grandiosity.

Examples of Grandiosity in Our Group

- All the name games when everyone gets a chance to present themselves. Just saying their name and giving themselves a last name that describes them, puts them on center stage for a minute.
- Whenever I do a double for someone in the group.
- All the vignettes-short psychodramas with role reversals.
- Whenever I simply ask someone for a response.

- Passing the pillow to a specific person
- Every time someone came up with a song.
- Whenever a new member joined the group, I would recommend that the participants ask that person something they would like to know about this new participant.

Moreno's Inspiration

Moreno's language, tools and techniques had a huge impact on the field of group psychotherapy. He developed a powerful way of treating people and is responsible for innovating methods for assessing a person's place in a group. He provided a framework where "you can practice living without being punished for making mistakes" (Karp, 1998, p. 3)

Moreno encouraged me to trust my instincts and trust the process. In his autobiography, Moreno recalls an encounter with Sigmund Freud in 1912.

> I attended one of Freud's lectures. He had just finished an analysis of a telepathic dream. As the students filed out, he singled me out from the crowd and asked me what I was doing. I responded, "Well, Dr. Freud, I start where you leave off. You meet people in the artificial setting of your office. I meet them on the street and in their homes, in their natural surroundings. You analyze their dreams. I give them the courage to dream again. You analyze and tear them apart. I let them act out their conflicting roles and help them to put the parts back together again."
>
> (Moreno, 1985)

Moreno Reflected

Moreno's writing is not easy to read. It is more beneficial to read what is written about him and his work, and I warmly recommend the books in the bibliography that talk about his theories and practice in order to learn more about this effective form of therapy. Antony Williams (1989) asserts:

> Psychodramas are like partisan plays: with apparent naturalism, they chronicle people's lives, deaths, loves, their hatred and suppression, their transcendence, their couplings and uncouplings. The other group members, the audience, discern in the psychodramatic narrative an echo of themselves. The plays are not finished products, like plays in a theatre, but poetic, dramatic works evolving on stage before the audience's eyes. . . . In psychodrama, the place of catharsis moves from spectator to the stage, to the actors themselves. Rare is the psychodrama where the audience is not moved as well: the catharsis becomes total, involving actors and audience. . . . People

who act out the situations – *protagonists* – express their phenomenal world outwardly in scenes, just as in a play. Honestly enacted psychodramas speak to our capacity for wonder and delight, to our sense of mystery and awe in our lives, arousing our sense of pity, beauty and pain, and fellowship with all creation.

(Williams, 1989, pp. 3–4)

Tian Dayton (1994, p. 7) says:

Psychodrama recreates the ordinary. It gives us the opportunity to say what was left unsaid and, in this way, to correct our original experience. It provides the pathway to bring our inner and outer reality into balance and accord. Society cannot always allow us to say what is in our hearts, but psychodrama can. It gives voice to our inner life, to the pain we are too ashamed to share, to the dream we hardly dare have.

Sharing My Process

I was used to ACTION in all of my work. I knew that it would be different at Melabev and it was, indeed. When I left the group after my first session, I cried. It was the kind of crying when your shoulders heave. I cried because the people were suffering from the worst loss of all – loss of their ability to connect. I cried because I couldn't reach them, though I had tried so hard. I cried because I was sure I would not be able to work with them. There was no eye contact, no smiles; there was no comprehension. I cried because it was so sad. I cried because I knew how the tools that I use always manage to help the groups I work with but here, I did not see how I could reach them, inspire them and move them to action and interaction. But I heard Moreno whisper to me "trust the process" and I did.

Throughout this book, I have been writing about the need for spontaneity and flexibility. Spontaneity is a basic mantra for Moreno. But more than my experience, spontaneity and skills, what happened here in my process was a deep inspiration to join, give, learn, expand and make it all work. This inspiration came from people who lived through difficult times and knew that no matter what, the choice is theirs. They had come to this center with the belief and hope that they could salvage their dignity no matter what. In every subject I brought to our sessions, they searched for the light, for the wisdom, for the strengths that helped them reach this age with large loving, loyal families.

An enormous help in their search was the use of narrative. In this process, I witnessed the need to tell our story somehow. I learned the value of narrative for this population. As Barbara Hardy states in her book: *An Approach Through Narrative,* (Durham University Press, 1968)

"We dream in narrative, remember, anticipate, hope, despair, believe, doubt, plan, revise, criticize, construct, gossip, learn, hate, and love by narrative." And yes, through DOING in drama, they have been able to generously share their insights, inner strengths and coping methods. They have found friendship, trust and the vitality to go on. As I have quoted from Tian Dayton, they did learn to speak the words they dared not speak but had shouting within them.

Summary of Practical Applications

- It is interesting and essential to read and understand the theoretical aspects of using psychodrama with this population. This section explains and gives practical examples of the application of concepts such as empathy, twinship, mirroring and grandiosity so that you will know WHAT to do and HOW to do, with a basic understanding of WHY.

- Understanding Heinz Kohut on a practical level, reading about my attitude towards his self-theory and meeting Moreno and understanding what he wanted to accomplish, produces more professional reliability and a more confident approach.

- After reading many examples and explanations of applying Moreno's tools, techniques and goals in group psychodrama, we can appreciate the need for creativity and spontaneity in our work.

Part VI

Coping With the Process

Meeting the Challenges

Dealing With Group Limitations and Adjustments

So far, I have mostly shared the success stories in our sessions. Many sessions were saved through flexibility and spontaneity on the spot. In this section, I want to discuss what didn't work and how that situation was handled. When this occurred, being flexible was to simply *accept* the limitations of many people in this group who were either too physically handicapped or cognitively impaired to respond. It was painful to admit that they could not carry out many basic instructions or that they just didn't get it – no way. Arriving at this acceptance was a major accomplishment for me. More important, accepting helped create new methods of working with this group. Here are a few examples of adjustments:

Organizing the Seating Arrangement: I have always found, in all my groups, that having criteria for where to sit in the circle – such as sitting according to your birthdate or the first letter of your name – helps integrate the members more quickly. Your neighbor on the left and on the right will more likely become your friend or at least develop some bond. With our group, this was impossible because too many members could not walk independently. I did, however, instruct the staff to try and have the members sit next to different neighbors as often as possible.

Feedback: I have a closing ceremony at the end of a session that I have made into a ritual with all of my other psychodrama groups. I ask the participants to share what they want to take from each session and what they would like to leave or throw away. I also have been using this closing ritual in my private practice. It is a subtle way of emphasizing the action insights of each session. The client does it and so do I. We each get a form of feedback. I always do this with my scarves so that we can *see* what we are taking and leaving from the session. It is

DOI: 10.4324/9781003321705-6

usually powerful and a reflection of the truth. In the first half year of work, some of the participants contributed to this closing ritual. Following are just a few examples which will show how much expression and sophistication we receive from this technique:

Jacob: I take the satisfaction, the good feeling from the true stories we heardtoday – emerald green. I want to throw away my negative prejudice and skepticism – purple.

Harvey: I take the memory of the fun we had today – green.
I want to throw away the lack of punctuality of the transportation to the Center – black.

Barbara: I take the encouragement to be honest – light blue.
I can't think of anything to throw away. (That was honest!)

Lionel: I take happiness, enjoyment – the session went very well indeed – red, orange, yellow. I want to throw away the bad mood from this past week – black.

Avi: I want to thank all of you for not saying no and for being so positive – orange. I want to throw away all the no's I managed not to say – black. (Avi was a very accomplished psychiatrist. He understood! He was a very active, wise participant until his condition deteriorated.)

Here is an example of what was said from another session without the use of the scarves.

Avi: I take that I have to remember to let go. I want to throw the black stuff that I had in my life.

Jacob: I take that everyone has different experiences but we can be reminded of our personal experiences. I want to throw away my uneasiness about my reactions to life experiences.

Barbara: I take the reminder to contact relatives. I want to throw away feeling alone.

Lilly: I can't forget what I want to forget and can't remember what I want to remember. I want to throw away my guilty conscience.

"I can't forget what I want to forget and can't remember what I want to remember."

From these examples, you can understand why it was so difficult for me to discontinue this ritual. Avi's Alzheimer's disease became progressively worse and he eventually left the center to go to another center where the spoken language was his mother tongue, Hebrew, and he did not have to live with the humiliation of his cognitive deterioration in front of the people in this group. Without him, I could no longer do this with our group, even without the scarves. There was too much resistance and not enough triggers every time I introduced this ritual at the end of our session. Believe me, I tried – too many times. Instead, sometimes *I* summarized what we could take and what we could leave from a specific session. This gave them feedback and summarized the session for them. If they, or the staff, had something to add, they contributed.

This method helped the participants remember and internalize what we had just dealt with in our session. For example, after our summertime session, I could say, "I take all the jingles and songs we remembered and just sang together. I leave the unbearable heatwaves we have been experiencing." I could also be more poignant and say at the close of a moving session. "I take your strength and hope and I leave your pain and frustration." Whenever I did this, many participants would nod their heads in agreement. They needed this summation of our sessions but I had to accept that they were incapable of organizing their thoughts and giving this form of expression to their experience. Yes, as you just read, it is much more powerful when it comes from them, but this was better than nothing at all. I still recommend that you try it at the end of your sessions. Every group responds differently.

The Scarves: Relinquishing the use of my scarves was not easy for me. They were my language for deep expression and concretization. There were two or three people in the group who did not like this tool. The resistance from this small group was infectious so I stopped using the scarves on a regular basis and saved them for special occasions. I always have my Mary Poppins bag filled with scarves whenever I go to work with a group. It is my warm-up to set them up on the table behind me. I need them. I love using them. This was a major relinquishment for me. They did not know what they were missing.

As you can see, in this case, accepting was more difficult because we did get valuable results from this tool. I learned that resistance is strong and contagious. I was actually surprised at how much expression we could achieve without the scarves. This was my most flexible switch in these five years. The people in the room noticed it and actually remarked appreciatively. After waiting a few years, I have occasionally brought the scarves back when I have felt that we need concretization with the help of the scarves, and the response has actually been positive.

The group now trusts my judgment. They have also enjoyed other props that I have brought to our sessions. They know that if I bring in my bag of scarves, there must be a good reason. Also, it is possible that they do not remember that they were once called my *schmattes*. Time and patience! But, more importantly, the group taught me that I can do psychodrama without my precious scarves.

Sociometry: We did *sociometric spectrograms* in their seats. In an ordinary psychodrama group, the participants place themselves on an imaginary line across the room from 1 to 10, according to how they feel about an issue that is brought up in the session. In our group, the participants raised their right hand, from 1 to 10 instead. If their response was #1, they placed their hand on their knee. They then would show by the distance from their knee, where they "stood" on this vertical hand scale. This adjustment actually became a helpful tool in all of my psychodrama Zoom sessions with all of my groups during the close-down due to COVID-19.

Role Reversal: I wanted the participants to experience being in the other role when a conflict was raised. For example, if one person was having trouble with his or her aide, I would ask that person to role reverse and be in the role of the aide. In the role, I would ask that person to tell me their name (as the aide), and tell me a little bit about the relationship with our client. I would get a lot of information from this role reversal and so would our client, who was actually providing the text. This is usually done by switching chairs. *Role reversing* was difficult for most of the participants physically and cognitively. They could not move from one chair to another easily. If they could, it took too long and it became arduous. As a result, I adapted how they performed role reversal with less need to move out of their chairs. I asked them to change the way they were sitting in the chair or do something symbolic so they would feel that they are in another role. Also, by my repeating what was just said, I helped them remember the text.

In most groups, the *protagonist* – the person who is working on this particular conflict or issue – looks around the room and picks someone who can portray the auxiliary ego. In our group, Michal or someone else on the staff would have to be the *auxiliary ego*, the other person being portrayed. Very rarely can we find someone in our group who is capable of being in the role and role reversing. Sometimes it is enough to ask them, "Who in our circle, would you choose to play a role or to play *you?*" Just selecting someone to represent you or a loved one is effective and therapeutic.

Closed group: Ideally, in order to build a cohesive group, we close the membership after the first few sessions. This was not possible. Our group and even our staff were very dynamic. All through these six plus years, I have had to regularly introduce new participants and new volunteers and find creative ways to incorporate them into our circle of trust.

Keeping distance: There is a rule in therapy that one does not disclose too much of one's personal life to the client. However, here I talked much more about my personal life than I would in any other group. My openness encouraged our participants to feel safe in revealing their personal information. It was a subtle but necessary invitation to them to open up, which they responded to.

Action: I accepted that the *action* in this group would be more verbal and stationary and less mobile. I learned that action can be achieved through subtle nuances.

Doubles: Being a double for someone who has just spoken was a regular and frequent occurrence. The participants loved when I did doubles for them but were resistant to do doubles for one another. It was too difficult for them. Standing behind a person, placing my hands on that person's shoulders and expressing what I felt he or she was feeling but not saying was always eagerly awaited by our group members. The double said the words that couldn't find a voice. The double expressed the sentences that were difficult to formulate. The double let loose the feelings that were deeply embedded in our participants' souls. The double gave voice to words that our participants needed to hear about themselves and their situations. It acted as a strong yet subtle form of validation.

When people in a group do doubles for one another, it creates a closeness of empathy and mutual trust. This group could not achieve this level of understanding and articulation. Who knows? If we continue working together, some participants could surprise me. I do occasionally ask, "Does anyone want to do a double for_____?" It has not happened yet!

Idiosyncrasies: When working with a psychodrama group, there are rules. We make a group contract where the issues deal with confidentiality, respect, commitment to the time schedule and issues like no cell phones. With this particular group, I actually successfully made a group contract at the very beginning of our process, at the request of one of our participants who was revealing a lot of personal information. We even used the scarves to sculpt the group contract so that they could *see* it. You can imagine how fulfilled I was! The words in the contract were theirs to own and see. Their contract was indeed unique. It assured them of confidentiality, honesty, openness, listening patiently, temperature control in the room, speaking loudly, no private conversations, loyalty, caring, togetherness, belonging, openness, warmth, action, spontaneity, truth, understanding, containment, respect and trust. These were all *their* words and ideas – and needs. We did have two psychotherapists in our group! They knew the language of support and contributed to this contract.

The reality was very different! The group was loyal to our contract. Everything that I mentioned above. It never dawned on me that we might need a few more rules like no pets, no guests, no eating, no leaving, no sleeping, and a lot more no's.

Carole needed to hold a pet in her lap. She also asked one of our volunteers to please bring *her* dog to our sessions. I am afraid of dogs but necessity is the mother and father of overcoming fear. Carole needed the softness of the pet in her lap and the security of having the volunteer's dog near her in order to feel comfortable in our circle. She was almost totally blind and very hard of hearing. This was her need and everyone was more than okay with it, including me. When was no small pet available, we found a soft cuddly puppet for her to hold.

Many of our participants would fall asleep and even snore loudly. This inappropriate behavior was usually caused by medication or insomnia. This recurring situation was treated with humor and slight nudges with the elbow. Also, no fuss.

Adrienne needed to knit or crochet. She brought a clunky bag filled with large needles and spools of wool. It became natural to hear the clinking of the needles and watch her work of art grow in front of our eyes.

Jacob was always late. There was no way to get him to the center on time. We all accepted this and somehow, we always managed to update him on what he had missed so that he could add his wise elucidations to whatever subject we were dealing with. He was needed and he knew it. His contributions to the discussions and actions were always inspiring and worth waiting for.

Susan needed space. She would suddenly get up and walk out of the room. Sometimes she would return and participate as if she never left. I never knew if or when she would return. She also missed many sessions.

Phones rang because our participants would forget to silence them. Sometimes we overheard personal conversations. Without making a fuss, we learned to remind and assist the people in shutting their phones.

Many times, some of our members did not manage to finish their breakfast before the beginning of our session. So, they ate during our session.

Whenever Lilly had a quote from Omar Khayyam, she would wait for a silent interlude in the session and start reciting it.

The dignity and *acceptance* within our group was such that no fuss was made over these discrepancies and no attention was paid to them. There was no need to include them in our distinguished contract. The idiosyncrasies became a part of our process, and I grew to love these exceptions to the rules because this illustrated who they were.

Here is a session that illustrates coping with group limitations:

After a Passover holiday vacation from the Center when we have not seen one another for two weeks, I like to bring an exercise that summarizes their experiences away from the comfort of our center. In a previous year, I had asked them to simply give a name or title to these two weeks, as if this period of time was a book or a film. Their responses were delightful and depicted so much truth. This exercise was in their comfort zone.

Lionel:	Dayenu! (Hebrew for enough)
Susan:	The greatest fun
Elaine:	Let them eat cake
Barbara:	*Balagan* (Hebrew for chaos)
Pauline:	The land of Nod
Marsha:	Weird
Lilly:	This year in Israel
Avi:	Freedom
Benjy:	Comedy times are here
Herbie:	What it means to be a husband on Pesach – the *schlepper* (Yiddish for the carrier, go-fer, runner.)
Simmy:	Not bad, pretty good

This past year, I thought that the members of this group were ready for something more sophisticated: *reflections.*

These are my instructions:

> "If you could give a name to a movie about your Passover holiday, what would you call it? Depict what this Passover was for you. Show us with your body and especially with your face."
>
> Up to here, the responses are ample.

As the session proceeds, it is apparent that my plan is beyond the capabilities of this group. I continue:

> Today we are going to do something we have never done before – *reflecting*. What was Passover for you? Don't say it, show it. Now everyone in the group, think, as if you were a *double*, and *reflect* back in a motion and expression what was feeling when he or she showed us what Passover was for him.

This is much too difficult for them! It might even be difficult for you, the reader to know what I am talking about. It is actually an exercise used to train *playback* troupes. When it works, it is a very effective group response. I might try it again. The one or two members who are able to reflect back on what they feel the person is trying to convey, do it quite well but more with words than with movement. This is not what I had planned, but it is still an accomplishment. Introducing the word reflecting gives our members a new tool for understanding others, and they are also exposed to new levels of a sophisticated form of communicating and connecting.

However, sometimes a session doesn't work at all! Yes, that can happen. We have high expectations of some magic taking place as a result of the exercises because that's what usually happens. Yet, sometimes it just doesn't work. The good news is that this is a diagnostic tool. We can learn from this situation. The truth surfaces loud and clear. Don't try to deny it, learn from it. And do what Moreno advised – be spontaneous. Some of our best sessions have evolved from moving from my plans to something new that evolved from their reactions.

Some of our best sessions have evolved from moving from my plans to something new that evolved from their reactions.

Dealing With the Difficulties of Dementia

Before I proceed with more detailed illustrations, I must add something that anyone who is dealing with this population will verify . . .

All of these descriptions of the dialogue in these sessions depict a group of elderly people who can respond appropriately with humor and vitality.

It is so easy to write up all these positive results but there were many times when |I looked at the group and saw a lot of blank faces. I saw faces sending a message of no, I can't. This is why this group was called the "Challenge Group". They were challenged in every way but they were also challenging me to help them rise out of the quicksand of old age and dementia diseases. They were challenging me to stimulate them to remember who they were and how rich and full their lives could still be. I was constantly reminded that many of the participants in this group have serious limitations, both cognitive and physical which I'm sure you realize after reading details of sessions. I would like to give you a better idea of the severity of the disease for these women and men.

The people in this group were not only dealing with issues of aging, Parkinson's and Alzheimer's disease, a few of the members in this group were coping with a more vicious form of dementia called Lewy bodies Dementia, the disease that drove Robin Williams, the famous actor and comedian, to commit suicide in 2014 at the age of 63. The difficulties for people in this group that I want to emphasize here range from:

- No control of parts of their bodies, including their bladders
- Difficulty in formulating sentences
- Constant shaking
- Serious hearing loss
- Serious vision impairment
- Constant pain
- Lack of balance
- Hallucinations
- Fatigue which leads to simply falling asleep in their seats
- Shame, frustration, anger, confusion, fear, embarrassment and depression
- Loss of self-confidence
- Not remembering even what was just said.
- . . . and much more.

Despite all of these barriers to successful group work, something happens in our circle that helps them overcome these impediments and interact with vitality. They forget their weaknesses as they discover their strengths via the group work. Being in their YES with total trust enforces positive functioning and overcoming genuine limitations. Their desire, curiosity, passion, memory and truth all emerge with a new strength and self-efficacy. We are aiming for and providing quality of life while dealing with the disease. Hopefully, through these forms of drama, we are succeeding in slowing down the trajectory of the disease.

Who Couldn't Stay in the Group?

The most difficult moments in this job were when I learned that the staff decided to transfer a participant to a lower functioning group because of a variety of reasons. The most obvious were connected to severe decline in cognition where the person was totally lost in our rich dynamic and challenging sessions.

One man had to leave because all of his responses had sexual innuendos. They were totally inappropriate for any group. He had no idea that his statements were morally offensive. In this case, it wasn't cognition issues, it was not having boundaries.

Another participant could not stop whistling. This was very annoying for all the people who had hearing aids. He could not control this because he was not really aware that he was whistling.

The saddest part was that afterward I would visit these former members of our group in the other rooms and they usually had no idea who I was. After building a relationship with a person through our process, it was devastating to witness this heartbreaking decline.

The knowledge that the person's cognition will eventually deteriorate is one of the most frightening aspects of dementia for all concerned. Our group was considered high functioning. I have tried to show you the limitations and challenges of working with this population. There is however a point where many of the activities designated for this group became too difficult for the members whose situations deteriorated. There were a few times that we held out as long as possible before transferring a group member because of the friendship that had developed between the members of our group. The men became pals. The women became close and comfortable with one another. These friendships were invaluable in producing a sense of kinship between all of the members.

I have used the words trust, safety, validation, identity, connecting and sharing numerous times when describing a rationale or a result of a session. These valuable assets were carefully measured against the declining cognition before anyone was transferred. For example, when our sweet member Herbie developed Lewy bodies Dementia, it was decided to keep him in the group, despite his hallucinations and confusion, because he felt so loved, protected and recognized for his humor, and affability in our circle. Once in a while, he would respond with an appropriate and even witty comment that made his presence precious and positive.

I must add here that I was not involved in deciding who must leave and who can stay in our group. The group leaders and the social workers of the staff had much more information on their situations. They frequently consulted with me. A major criterion became, if they can function appropriately in the psychodrama sessions, then they are capable of staying in this group.

Dealing With the Loss of a Group Member

There were at least ten losses in our group in these past five-plus years. Sadly, the *only* advantage of memory loss is that when a member of our group no longer comes to our sessions, the others do not miss this person. Also, I discovered that the word *death* or *died* does not scare our participants. It is a natural part of life for them. I suppose when you are 93 or 98, you see things differently!

We would tell the group the sad news and then move on. There were times when the death of a member deeply affected the participants and there was a need for group therapy. When I felt the need for processing, psychodrama was very helpful. Since our members could not physically or probably even cognitively pay a condolence call to that person's family, I would put an *empty chair* in the center of the circle and say:

> Let's pretend that we are going to pay a condolence call to our deceased friend's family. Seated in this chair is a member of his family. What would you like to say about our dear friend who just passed away? Tell that family member some of the special things you know about our dear lost friend.

And, of course, they did – gladly, without any hesitation. They were familiar with this tool and were able to use it to recall their fond memories of their dear friend who was no longer with us. One time, I was daring and actually asked them to tell the group what *they* would want people to say about *them* after they pass away. This is a form of *future projection*. Again, they were able to respond openly and freely. That particular session actually made them think about how they would like to be remembered and led to some determination. I could see it in their eyes and feel it in the energy in the room and I gave it a few group doubles: *I now realize that I am so loved. Or: Perhaps I should change the way I react to certain people before it is too late.* Their heads were nodding in agreement.

My personal double here should be: *I really should have called this section "Dealing With Death" but that word was too stark for me.*

Now that I have delineated the challenges of working with this group, I am sure you will be moved by this next segment which brings the responses of professionals who work closely with this population.

Summary of Practical Applications

- Everyone who deals with this population needs flexibility and spontaneity.
- The idiosyncrasies, the deterioration in functioning and the natural dynamics of this age group must be handled gently and wisely.
- Humor and lightness are helpful as well.
- You are not only the facilitator, you are the resilient, protective symbol of strength and continuity. Your group will inspire you, and you must always be ready for the unknown.

> You are not only the facilitator, you are the resilient, protective symbol of strength and continuity.

Training People Who Work With the Elderly

As a result of doing psychodrama at the Melabev Center, I have been asked to give workshops to professionals who work with this population. I would like to share their perception of the elderly with you which will enrich what I have been describing. My sessions are seventy-five minutes a week. These professionals, mostly social workers, spend much more time with the elderly and deal directly with their daily lives.

When I asked the participants in these workshops to sculpt a senior citizen with the scarves, these were their honest, sensitive, experienced descriptions (Image 6.1):

- Stubborn
- Soft
- A treasury of wisdom
- Transparent
- Very needy
- Lonely
- Complicated but colorful
- Been there, done that – yes full of experience
- Despondent
- Dignified
- A history with strong roots
- Needs support
- Nuisance
- A lot of knowledge
- Opinionated
- Helpless

- Weak
- Full of pain
- Frustrated
- Anxious and afraid of everything
- Forgetful
- Spiritual
- Sick
- Threatened
- Afraid of change
- Feeble

After the group of professionals sculpted "The Golden Age", I asked *them* to *be* the senior citizens, through role reversal, and tell these trained caretakers, whatever they wanted and needed for them to know. The responses illustrated how connected these therapists were with their clientele, and can give you important information. Here is what they said in their role as the elderly:

"I'm alive."
"I am vital!"
"Help me remember who I am."
"There are a lot of things that bother me."
"I am full of love and softness beneath this exterior."
"I don't want to feel left out."

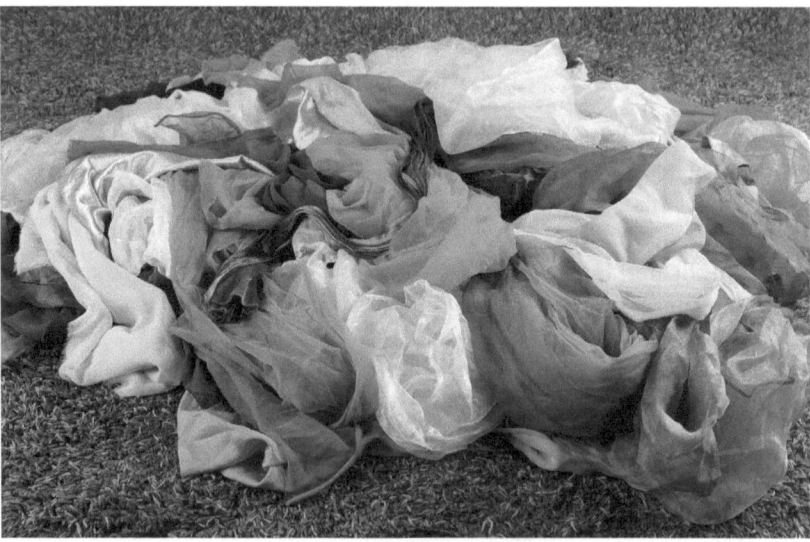

Image 6.1 The "Golden Age", as seen in the eyes of people training to work with this population

"Thank you for listening."
"Don't tell my children."
"Help me."
"I've had enough."
"You are saving my life."
"Please don't forget about me."
"When will I see you again?"
"You make me feel so good."
"Don't leave me."

And, of course, "Who are you? What do you want? Why are you here?"

In these workshops, I could feel the devotion and total involvement of the professionals with the elderly, but more importantly, I could see how rewarding and satisfying working with the elderly can be.

Summary of Practical Applications

Reading about the training of geriatric social workers is a window to what is facing you.

Two methods used with these workers are:

1. Sculpt a senior citizen in order to create awareness.
2. Have the social workers role reverse with the people they work with in order to create empathy.

Part VII

Adapting the Process

Dealing With New Situations: Creating a Psychodrama COVID-19 Zoom Group

The advent of the COVID-19 pandemic changed everything. Our welcoming happy center was closed. In order to avoid the effects of isolation and lack of stimulation, something had to be done – from the homes. The staff used resourcefulness and invited all of the clientele to meet on Zoom.

The following section will be very detailed because this was all new and experimental. Yes, it was an unexpected part of this process. Fortunately, these sessions were recorded so that we could analyze them. I am writing it in a diary form to describe my planning process and then the reality of what worked and what was totally different. I am adding this important part in the hope that it will encourage you, the reader, to never say never. Who would have thought that elderly people with dementia could connect, communicate and care on Zoom? Who would believe that we can do drama, in many of its forms, on Zoom? Who would have thought that when the center reopened, we would miss the Zoom sessions and the unique opportunity to meet our participants in their home environment and meet their partners, aides, and see photo collages and other significant items in their homes? Who would have believed that you can reach out and touch someone on a screen?!

> . . . Never say never. Who would have thought that elderly people with dementia could connect, communicate and care on Zoom . . . ? Who would have believed that you can reach out and touch someone on a screen?!

Plans and Implementation

April 16, 2020

This was my biggest challenge at Melabev, so far. Due to the COVID-19 lockdown, Melabev has offered our members two Zoom sessions a day.

DOI: 10.4324/9781003321705-7

One is a music session in the morning and the other one, at four in the afternoon, is a yoga session or a lecture of some sort or more often another music session. In these sessions, the audience is mostly passive. Most of the people who join in are not from our group. Their functioning is on a lower level than the group I work with.

I was called upon to conduct a session on the day that Israel commemorates the Holocaust. This day is called *Yom Hashoah* – Holocaust Memorial Day. It certainly is a day where upbeat music is not appropriate. It is befitting for me to DO something with the people at Melabev on this day and help the participants give expression to all the emotions flooding their souls.

As I have written throughout this book, I *DO*! Well, what does a psychodrama therapist *DO* on Zoom on this intense and sensitive day? How can I help everyone feel relevant? How do we handle the mute and unmute? And, what can I do that is appropriate for the diverse levels of the participants? I have to deal with the contents of this session and make sure I have their attention. I have to respect the subject we are dealing with, the physical and cognitive limitations of our participants, the needs for connection, stimulation and validation and this new method of getting together.

Thankfully, Nancy Brown, the staff member hosting all the Zoom sessions, would be taking care of all the technical aspects. This was a big relief for me. She runs all of the sessions and is adept and unbelievable with the people. She runs the room with the people who are at the lowest cognitive level. I love to watch her work with them whenever I come to the Melabev center. Her energy is so positive and enabling. When I observed Nancy, on the screen sitting in front of her computer, all bespectacled, I actually did not realize she was the same zany incredible leader in our center! Knowing that she was in charge was very reassuring. The fact that Jennie, our devoted, sensitive and very professional leader in our Challenge Group would also be participating and helping with the unmuting and noticing who needed to speak and worrying about all the needs of each person in her group, was heartening and encouraging. And, of course, Jackie our devoted social worker, Dvora the excellent director of our center and Chariklia, our prodigious resident medical consultant, would also be there to contribute in their inimitable ways. They are each and all an inspiration and so attuned to the needs of all the participants. I am glad I just had a chance to mention just a few of the special people who work at the center and who have become cherished friends. Knowing that these capable staff members were on board would enable me to deal with the content of our session and my attempts to use psychodrama in order to reach and benefit as many participants as possible. Yes, this would definitely be teamwork. I also hoped that Michal, our incredible volunteer who contributes so much in our sessions at the center, as an *auxiliary ego*, playing all the roles in our role reversals would eventually be able to help me develop some psychodramatic interactions.

This was all new and there is definitely an excitement in trying something different and having no idea how it would turn out. Actually, the following sessions became my introduction and internship for all of my work as a psychodrama therapist during the pandemic.

> This was all new and there is definitely an excitement in trying something different and having no idea how it would turn out.

These are some of the issues I wanted to relate to:

- I have never conducted a Zoom session.
- This is a very large group of people.
- Our lives have totally changed because of this terrible pandemic.
- Our children and grandchildren cannot visit us.
- We cannot leave our homes.
- Actually, we are seeing everyone in their homes!
- Many of us are feeling isolated and confused.
- We have to cope with new challenges.
- I need to create a safe and secure circle of trust for the participants.
- Some of the people might feel intimidated by Zoom.
- There could be many unpredictable technical intrusions in our sessions.
- It is difficult to connect emotionally on Zoom but it is possible.
- Some people are embarrassed in front of a camera.
- I need to find ways to encourage spontaneity on the screen.
- I want to enable and foster validation and connection – on the screen.
- When someone responds to a question, the others can achieve a sense of social cohesion; gain this essential feeling of "us" and instill the feeling of I am not alone, I belong.
- It is essential to encourage communication with others on the screen in order to empower them through identification with others. I want them to gain new options from one another.
- I need to teach the participants the new rules on Zoom.
- It is not easy for them to figure out how to be seen and how to see others. It can be extremely confusing.
- People can enter and leave. This can be very distracting.
- Holocaust Remembrance Day is a daunting day.
- People who had to cope with the Holocaust and survived could inspire and contribute. We still have people like that in our groups.

Over the years we have heard many stories about their fleeing from Europe to the United States, Canada or England during the Holocaust.

- We would want to know how others are coping.
- There are many songs that can inspire and evoke the proper atmosphere. I will listen till I find the perfect song and the most appropriate rendition.

What you just read were my needs. Now I needed to consider the needs of the participants. If I had to participate in a Zoom session on this serene and serious Day of Remembrance, what would I need from this session?

- I would want to feel a sense of *twinship*, belonging.
- I would want to hear how others are coping.
- I miss being with the people I can see on the screen.
- I am filled with emotions that I need to express, explore and share.
- I am nervous about the technical aspects of participating in a Zoom session.
- Will I be able to hear?
- Will everyone hear me?
- Will they see me?
- I am also nervous about my condition. Will I understand what is being said and done? Will I remember who everyone is? Will they remember me? Will I feel lost?
- Will it be interesting or boring?
- How do I feel about sharing my Melabev world with my family or with my aide?
- How do I feel about sharing my family with my Melabev world?

Yes, there are a lot of new factors to take into consideration for the participants as well as for myself.

Zoom Sessions

Plans and Implementation

I plan my first Zoom session.

I will open the subject by telling the participants on the screen how in terror situations the families are alone in their terrible loss and pain. Everyone else can go on with their lives. In the Holocaust, half of the world was suffering. For the rest of the world, life had not changed significantly. But now, with the COVID-19 pandemic, everyone in the world is in the same situation. Everyone!

What are we feeling?

I can show them my emotion cards and they will raise their hands if they are feeling these emotions. We can talk about them. Another option could be to discuss what do we DO in order to cope?

I will tell the story of when I worked with Second-Generation Holocaust survivors. I asked them to bring an object – real or psychodramatically – that could tell about their parents who had survived the Holocaust.

One woman in the course brought in tweezers. Her mother managed to sneak it into the concentration camp. She hid it behind the toilets, in her barracks, knowing no one would ever clean there. Yes, she used them to tweeze her eyebrows and maintain a sense of humanity and dignity.

Another woman brought in a beautifully embroidered white tablecloth. It was her dowry. Her grandmother, who did not survive, had it specially embroidered for her daughter's dowry. The grandmother buried it near a tree, hoping to retrieve it after the war. Fortunately, her mother did find it when she returned to her small village. She pulled it out of its deep burial place and to her astonishment, it was pure white and clean as could be. The earth had protected it.

I'd like to share about myself, that maybe it is vanity or maybe it is something much deeper, but here in our isolated COVID-19 world where I see no one but my darling husband every day, I still make sure I like what I see when I look in the mirror in the morning. Why? It is in order to still be ourselves. I want to see that person who usually goes out to work, who goes to the gym, who visits her grandchildren. I want to be me at my best – even if it is only between me and myself! So, I get dressed nicely every morning. I fix my hair and do my eyebrows. Yes. I must do these things if I want to be in touch with my own humanity. It is not vanity. No, it is humanity.

This sharing about myself acts as a trigger for them to open up. Most of the participants are not in our psychodrama group and do not know the language and do not trust me or the method . . . yet.

To strengthen this theme, I will find a short story about an object in the Holocaust. Elie Wiesel wrote a story called "The Watch" based on the same idea but with a different ending. I will edit the story and prepare a dramatic reading of it for them. After the reading, I will ask them what objects would we bring to tell about how we are surviving this difficult time. I will give them some examples.

> A woman showed her grandmother taking out her old, very used sewing machine. The grandmother is sewing beautiful masks, from fabric that she has, to be donated for use in this COVID-19 crisis.
> The fridge – our favorite place to visit.
> The iPhone – to connect via WhatsApp.
> The computer for all the Zoom sessions.

The TV, photo albums of the family.
Now we will be ready to delve deeper.

Many people in this population can't help but make comparisons between the Holocaust and this COVID-19 pandemic. But there are many differences: Firstly, we are NOT hungry. No one is starving because of COVID-19. We might be alone physically but we are very connected via our phones and computers and TVs. This is very helpful to our emotional health. We have a strong Jewish country that is taking care of us. The entire world is fighting the same enemy.

After this thought process, I write out my program to make sure this will run smoothly. I never do this precision work for my live sessions with my group. With a session on Zoom I feel I must be very organized. I am not working alone here. There are at least five staff members attending who will help recognize the raised hands, but I should have a precise plan in order for this session to run smoothly. This is an outline of my program:

Zoom Sessions

Program
Hello – to everyone on gallery view – 5 minutes
I must start with my own personal blessing – called *Shehechiyanu*, a prayer we say when experiencing something for the first time in the year.
I say this prayer because I have never led a psychodrama or any kind of session on Zoom before and this special blessing is for something new in our lives, "Blessed art thou . . . that we have lived and have existed and have reached this time."
This is *our* Holocaust day ceremony.
Almost every Holocaust day ceremony starts with this song.
"Eli Eli" (The Road to Caesarea) – 2 minutes
Read Wikipedia about this song – 3 minutes
Share my thoughts on the situation – 2 minutes
Ask: What are we feeling?
This is an emotional day and these are emotional times.
There are so many different emotions that we are feeling.
I made cards of many of our emotions. I will read them to you and you can raise your hands if you are feeling any of these emotions – even the relatives and aides watching with you can participate and share – 10 to 20 minutes.
Tell the story of when I worked with Second-Generation survivors. And lead up to Eli Wiesel's story, "The Watch" – 7 minutes
Dramatic reading of the story – 15 minutes

What objects would we bring to show and tell about how we are surviving this difficult time? Give examples as a trigger – 10 minutes.

Finale: Screenshare with the Koolulam Video of Holocaust survivors
and three Generations singing the song "Chai" (Alive) – 5 minutes

Closing: Unmute everyone so they can chat and say goodbye till the
next Zoom.

This *was* my plan!

Now I will write about what actually happened in this experimental Zoom
session. Seeing and meeting all the people in their squares on Zoom was
indeed overwhelming. I knew only the people from my group but I had
to relate to all of them. There were people lying, almost lifeless, in their
bed. There were people being handled and assisted by their aides or
families. Some people were eating. Others were half asleep. But, many of
them were waiting eagerly for something – anything – to happen.

Zoom Session # 1

Implementation

Something happened to me at the moment that I finished my quick
scan. There were over seventy participants. I had to embrace all of them.
There was something in the screen that propelled me. There was this tre-
mendous and deep need to pull all of those people in boxes together and
make one group. I forgot about my detailed and very well-prepared program. I looked at them. I gave instructions and they followed through:
"Everyone – take your hands and give yourself a good hug." We all need
that. They did.

> I spontaneously continued with what had to follow.
> "Let's form our Zoom Group right here.

Now . . . everyone put your arms out as far as they can go in order
to reach everyone on this zoom and we will create a giant hug." They
understood and they did it. They also needed these hugs. It was so obvious. And then I said: "Yes, now we are all together!" They understood.
They felt it. They knew it. I was feeling at home!

I then introduced the song that would open our ceremony. I asked
them to raise their hands if they knew of Hannah Szenes, the writer of
the poem that formed the lyrics of this song. To my surprise, quite a
few raised their hands. I read out the English translation of the words.
Nancy, the group host, then showed them the YouTube of the song and
everyone – well mostly everyone – listened. It is a beautiful arrangement
sung by a girls' choir. You have to be moved by the mesmerizing melody
and the power of the words.

I then did my program as planned but asked them to raise their hands as often as possible. When I asked them how many of them were Holocaust survivors, only two or three replied. There were definitely more but they were not able to remember or were not concentrating on my question. I was not surprised. But, throughout the rest of the session, we discovered many more first- and second-generation survivors. After the story, there were a few appropriate responses to my question about objects that could tell about them.

I then turned to the emotion cards. I had planned to work with many conflicting emotions that would help them express their frustration, fears and loneliness but it just did not feel right. Instead, I talked about the cacophony of emotions we are all feeling and instinctively showed them the card with the word PROUD. I asked them to raise their hands if they wanted to share something that they are proud of. There were wonderful responses. Yes, they have so much to be proud of. Most of them were proud of their families and rightly so. When Deena talked about her family and expanded on how they were artists and accomplished people and started raving about them with a big smile. I replied, "Deena you should also be proud of your amazing smile. Whenever you smile, it brings magic." And, of course, her smile grew. I told her that today with COVID-19 everything is contagious. I asked her to move her face close to the screen and give us her best biggest smile so that we could all catch it from her. I then asked everyone to move their faces closer to the screen so that they could catch Deena's smile. And they did. Her smile proved to be very contagious. Almost all of them were smiling. But over and beyond the buoyant participation, something happened to Deena. Instead of being a passive listener, all curled up under a blanket, physically distant from the screen, she blossomed into an inspiring giver of warmth and vitality. This was a prime example of *grandiosity*.

I then showed them the card with the word APPRECIATION and one man told us how much he appreciated his wife. I am sure she was smiling! We had more replies but no one was documenting in my blue notebook and I don't remember what was said. I do remember though that they did respond with enthusiasm. The other participants listened intently.

This was an experiment and the people reacted. Even through the screen, we sensed that they felt a part of something, a part of a nation, a part of the Melabev family and a part of this particular first Zoom psychodrama session. I was exhausted but so moved!!! I was asked to continue.

Zoom Session #2

April 28, 2020

For Israel Independence Day I already knew there would be over seventy participants from all of the groups. In this Zoom session, I wanted total immersion and involvement in something we all have in common, the celebration of our national holiday.

I wanted to create a group experience through creative dramatics where we can make anything happen. I wanted them to learn that:

- We can behave *as if.*
- We can pretend.
- We can take a flight of fantasy and simply celebrate this special day together because in drama anything is possible!

Opening Ritual

I officiate by saying: Give yourself a hug because you are here with us at Melabev Zoom and we can't give you one so, make it happen.

Now stretch your arms to reach everyone and let's make a group.

You all lived through the Shoah (Holocaust) but you also lived through the birth of our State of Israel.

Do any of you remember when the State was born?

Where were you when Ben Gurion announced that we have a state?

We must celebrate together. We cannot go out and be with our friends and family but we here can be a Melabev family and celebrate this important holiday together. So, let's start with "*Erev Chag*" (the eve of the holiday – most Jewish holidays begin the night before). Every year there is a torch bearing ceremony which is a transition from Yom Hazikaron, Remembrance Day, to Yom Haatzmaut – Independence Day.

Let's celebrate. We will begin with the Torch Lighting ceremony. How many of you have ever seen this beautiful ceremony? It is very special. Let's watch it for one minute. Below is what is written on the screen. I read it out.

- The annual ceremony is held at Mount Herzl in Jerusalem.
- It is attended by distinguished guests of State from all over the world and 5,000 citizens
- But this year things will be a little different. COVID-19 has forced a rethink on the ceremony. Without losing this national tradition.
- For the first time ever, there will be no audience.
- The entire ceremony will be livestreamed.
- The climax is the lighting of the twelve torches symbolizing the twelve tribes of Israel that are selected by a specially elected committee.
- To be selected as a torchbearer is a great honor
- The ceremony is watched by millions in Israel and all around the world.

I proceed: Let's think. Who would *you* choose to light a torch? I'll tell you who I am choosing!

I choose each and every one of you.

Yes.

And this year you are all going to light a torch for *your* contribution to our Jewish world.

You all are so strong. You are not giving up.

You come to Melabev to enrich your lives. You have built beautiful families. You are all so very brave. You all moved to Israel. You are working hard to continue. It is not easy but you are doing it. So, everyone, take a torch. Hold it up high with pride and dignity. You know who you are. You know what you have done in your life and you certainly know how you are coping today – by being here and making this ceremony happen.

Now, together, let's light the light. Everyone say, I am – say your name, (the son or daughter of, with your mother's name and your father's name). For some of them, this is a challenge. But the magnet is working and everyone is holding a torch in their right hand.

I continue: Now we will all say, I – (say your name) am lighting this torch for the glory of the Land of Israel.

Who else can we choose to light a torch?

Think of someone who has overcome difficulties.

Think of someone who has made a distinct contribution to the State of Israel.

The participants actually asked the people on the staff to light a torch for the marvelous devoted work they do at our center. This was a chance for them to honor the people who take care of them for so many hours of their challenging week. It was empowering for them. It was a way to give expression to so many emotions.

I continue: Now let's have some fireworks. We are all going to be the fireworks. Let's watch a minute of fireworks and then all of you get ready to BE the fireworks. Our ceremony is going to have everything.

Did you ever see the fireworks at the ceremony at Mount Herzl, in Jerusalem? Raise your hand if you did. Well, we are going to make some right now. Everyone put on your brightest lights and let them fly through the air to impress everyone. Use your hands in every way possible to be the fireworks. This is a first. We can make fireworks right here but you have to help me. We even have appropriate background music for our fireworks.

I then proceed with my plan. I say: What am I proud of in Israel? The IDF – The Israel Defense Force. Let's go out and see our great army. Let's salute them and celebrate them. We will now watch a YouTube video about the different divisions of our army.

What else can we do to celebrate? FOOD every Jewish celebration must have food! What's a Jewish Holiday without FOOD??

Now let's make our *mangal*. Who knows what a *mangal* is? It is our barbecue. What should we eat? Now let's talk about *Atzmaut* – Independence. Last year our group did an exercise where we gave Israel an imaginary gift. We can do that in drama. All of these *gifts* were documented in my blue book. I will read them to you now. This is what you gave to Israel a year ago.

Herbie:	Prosperity
Monica:	light
Lila:	A donation
I say:	Now let's add to this list today.
Staff:	everyone should listen to everyone, politeness, new immigrants, pride, water, respect for people, values, heritage. (This was a good trigger and the participants responded well.)
Brian:	Victory
Lila:	Hope
Mitch:	Strength and devotion
Deena:	Trees
Lionel:	Leadership
Benjy:	To be tough
Barbara:	Growth in nature

What gift have I received from Israel?

Libby:	Being home
Mitch:	My grandchildren
Adrienne:	Inspiration
Barbara:	Joy and care for the elderly.
Monica:	Hope and National Pride
Deena:	Being a part of building – my son built a *yishuv*, a community in Israel.
Shoshana:	A sense of security
Manny:	A large family
Martin:	Pride in our innovation and our brains.
Lionel:	My home!
Brian:	Freedom
Lila:	Renewal of hope for the future.
Others add:	Water, prosperity, light, good health, continuity, a sense of belonging and new beginnings.

We will end with a very special Koolulam video featuring 12,000 people, including Israel's President Reuven Rivlin, singing a very popular Israeli song, *Al Kol Ale* (For All These) by Naomi Shemer.

> OF STING AND HONEY
> By Naomi Shemer
> (English version: Naomi Shemer)
> All the stings and all the honey
> All the wrongs and all the right
> And our little baby daughter –
> Need your leading light
> Keep the water pure and flowing

Keep the fires lively warm
There's a murmur slowly growing
Toward a distant home
We are praying, we are praying
For the close ones we adore
Listen to our silent crying
Deepest sorrows – fears of war
Don't uproot the newly planted
Give me hope and hold my hand
Lead me homeward, lead me safely
To my blessed promised land.

Conclusions From This Session

Because this was a large diversified group, it was necessary to prepare a detailed program for this session. The action here was mostly group work. However, when I asked who they think deserved to light a torch, three people raised their hands and gave the torch to three people on the staff. The participants treasured being a part of an official ceremony. They heard the glory in the language and felt the nobility (*grandiosity*).

They all moved their hands together with lots of energy and gusto in order to make the fireworks (*twinship*). The members of my group loved hearing their names singled out mirroring their responses three years ago when I read out what they had said so long ago. In essence, the Zoom Group used drama in a group experience to celebrate this national holiday in the traditional way.

The sessions I have just described were ceremonies with over seventy people. I was the officiator. Our next session will be a totally different experience. The staff and I will build a small group where we can concentrate on more involvement and expression from them and less from me, and here I will be the facilitator.

Zoom Session # 3

May 5, 2020

Participants: A smaller group. This time only the members of the Challenge group including members who do not come on Tuesdays and three people from the lowest level group who I thought would be able to give and to receive in this small group. There were twenty-six participants (one screen), which included five staff members. The purpose of this session was:

- To create a group, of higher functioning people with dementia, where the tools of psychodrama will facilitate interaction on a Zoom screen.

- To create a safe space filled with trust and possibility.
- To create a space both intimate and dynamic.
- To facilitate connection and identity.
- To achieve *empathy, twinship, mirroring, and grandiosity* on a screen. (See section on Kohut for these terms.)
- To use sociometry in order to attain options, identification and validation and a social experience.

Before starting I had to consider a few important objective facts: The participants are technically dependent on their aides or family members. Some of them do not have computers. Their iPhone or iPad screens do not project everything and everyone. A few of them are not living in their usual familiar settings. They have moved in with children or grandchildren. Some of them cannot hear. Some of them cannot see. Some of them are confused and disoriented. Some of them are experiencing depression due to a new kind of social isolation. Some of them cannot remember from session to session and even from moment to moment. Some of them do not recall who the other people are. Some of them have no idea who I am and what I do. Some of them need an explanation of what psychodrama, the Theater of Truth, and role reversal are. Some of them have no idea what I *do* with the groups. Most of their Zooms are with people who sing familiar songs to them. I have no piano or other musical instruments.

I open with a ritual for grounding. We start out with our opening ritual of hugging ourselves so that we can feel the warmth, affection and closeness that we all are feeling when we see each other. I then tell them to reach out, as far as their hands could stretch to try and caress everyone so that we can have one big holding. I was speaking in *their* language.

In order to give everyone a feeling of belonging (*twinship*), a sense of identity and individual attention at the same time (*grandiosity*), I ask everyone to announce their names and add an adjective that describes them. I make it clear that I really want to get acquainted with all of them, especially one-third of the group who are new to me. They take this very seriously. Jennie sends me an alphabetical list of the participants. Everyone participates and everyone listens with interest and respect. I use the tool of *sociometry* to measure how much they identify with each adjective by telling them:

- Raise your right hand up to the top of the screen if you also have this trait.
- Raise your right hand up to the middle of the screen if you have this trait moderately.
- Lower your right hand to below the screen if you do not have this trait.

They do it each time. There are a few times that I have to remind them to *show* us. I give them a few examples and *show* them. Thank you, Moreno!

This is an action that the participants can do. It makes them feel social cohesion.

These are their descriptive adjectives:

Adrienne – animated and she was animated when she said it
Brian – loving, talkative
Bill – powerful
Barbara – optimistic
Deena – lovable
Geoffrey – anxious by nature, companionable
Herbie – curious
Harvey – emotional
Hannah – nice, honest, family person, grandchildren person
Lila – loving, inquisitive
Leah – honest, keeps the mouth shut
Morty – introvert
Moe – intelligent
Malka – friendly
Mitch – *quacker*
Shneur – helpful
Shoshana – patient
Susan – care for other people
Gila – upbeat
Nancy – outgoing
Me – spontaneous, flexible
Miriam Stein – coping
Jackie – giving
Jennie – caring, bossy

I would like to point out that I made a few interventions that were impulsive and actually worked. When I said hello to Herbie who is having a very hard time concentrating and connecting, I asked him what color were his socks. His cognition has deteriorated tremendously due to the progression of his Lewy Bodies disease. He always wears very bright glowing socks in our sessions. This has become his trademark. This question helped him associate what was happening on the screen with his life at the Melabev center and the people on the screen.

Also, Harvey was no longer in our Tuesday group. I felt a need to connect to him personally after not seeing him for two years. When I met Harvey on the screen, I commended him on the book he had published a year ago. This was a risk but it did the trick. The staff commented after the session that they have not seen him so happy (*grandiosity*) in a very long time. This interaction gave him the courage and the will to participate.

I let Lila know that, by using the adjective "inquisitive" she had given me an option. I would try to be more inquisitive. Everyone should also think what trait could they could adopt for themselves? When Jennie read out the list of adjectives, they experienced audio mirroring of what they had said, not to mention a reminder! I asked them to listen and think which traits would be beneficial for them in the way that I had related to being inquisitive.

When I asked them to show us who else is bossy, by raising their hands, three of the participants pointed to their spouses who were nearby. Herbie's wife came on and pointed to him! Humor is always helpful! Libby pointed to her daughter-in-law and Bill pointed to his wife. I thanked Jennie for introducing the word bossy. We had never really explored that word. In one of our future sessions, I will start with a sentence: I am bossy when and . . . when I am bossy . . .

Bossy is something we say about others. We don't admit that we are bossy but bossy can be a positive thing when we want to pursue what we know is right.

When I asked what descriptive adjective would you like to give to one another, (connection) one woman spoke about her friend and said she is "wonderful". She introduced a word that intrigued me and which I decided to amplify as follows. Wonderful! What a wonderful description. But we don't usually say that about ourselves. Somebody else says it about us. I want you all to think – who would say that you are wonderful. Think about all the people you know. They were all smiling with acknowledgment but no one volunteered. Albeit there was an abundance of positive energy in our "zoom room" I decided to pursue this further. I gave them homework. Who would think I am wonderful?

I will start the next session with checking their homework and if necessary, asking their families and aides to help them give their answers. I might meet them through role reversal and ask them WHY they think our participant, in our group, is wonderful.

I will move on to the adverb: wonderfully! We can say that we sing wonderfully. What else do we do wonderfully? This will give them a much-needed sense of worthiness. This will help them hug themselves in this COVID-19 time when there are no opportunities for physical contact and expressions of love.

Summary

When this session was over, I was not exhausted. I was exhilarated. I did not have to work hard in order to reach them. They were eager and ready for action. They needed it. They wanted it and they got it!

I realized something very significant. I am now really excited about our Zoom sessions. I will have to make serious adjustments and find new ways to adapt the tools and techniques that you have been reading about, so that I can help the participants achieve vitality, identity and meaning, but I am no longer threatened by the screen and the distance. I actually felt very close to them and afterward, in reviewing the session with the staff, we saw a screen filled with people who were smiling, animated and connecting. We saw people who would benefit from psychodrama on Zoom.

Zoom Session #4

May 13, 2020

I will proceed by just describing new information on dealing with the challenges and fulfillment of using Zoom with our population.

In this session, I try a new form of creating *twinship, grandiosity* and *mirroring* through sound. I make it my business to let them hear their names as often as possible and clap their hands or stamp their feet frequently.

After our opening ritual, I ask, "Who would say you are wonderful?" For example, Bill answers, "Who thinks I am wonderful? My wife!" His wife, Mabel, who is on the screen sitting right next to him, gives us a thumbs up.

I then proceed bravely and attempt a role reversal. I say to Bill, let's pretend you are Mabel, "What would you say if you were Mabel?" His reply shows that he has not understood what I wanted. He is not a member of our Tuesday group but he is in the Challenge group on other days.

Bill's first response is, "I appreciate Mabel very much." When I repeat my instructions and say, "Make believe YOU are Mabel", he replies with wit and humor, "That's a very difficult job." I repeat, "If you were Mabel, what would she say about you?" He quickly says, "That I am kind and respectful. That I am a good person." I feel so glad that I didn't give up. I proceed, "Mabel, since you are here, tell us, was he telling the truth?" She replies, "Oh he is minimizing it. He is so much more than that. He is funny. He uses his humor to make everyone around him happy. He likes to hear people laugh and be happy. That's his best trait." Bill is glowing. This exercise just got better and better as we heard wonderful things about our members through role reversals.

I then experiment with sound by asking them to stamp their feet to chase the COVID-19 away. All through the session, instead of showing with their hands, I ask them to clap their hands instead to express their connection through sound. I discover very quickly that this form of connection through sound does not work well on Zoom. When I invite each person to have a solo and say goodbye to whoever they choose on the screen, the response is full of positive energy.

Zoom Session #5

May 20, 2020

For the following session I had planned a surprise birthday party with all the trimmings for our beloved group leader, Jennie. Here is a brief summary of the program:

I say: Today is someone's birthday. Do you know who?

HAPPY BIRTHDAY TO JENNIE
Please sing along with this video. I want to hear you. UNMUTE
We have a few special guests who would not miss this for the world.
Sit back as we celebrate you today.
Listen to this song, "You've Got a Friend". I am sure that everyone
on this screen will agree that you are always there for every single
one of us. You think of everything and you are there wherever and
whenever we need you.
This is what you are for me. I know you are always there to understand
me and I am sure that everyone in the group feels the same way!
(Play "You've Got a Friend".)
Now we can really take advantage of the fact that you are all at
home. We can give a blessing and even give her a gift from our
homes. I have an object in my home that I want to use to tell you
what I want to give to you and what I want to tell you on your
birthday. It is a plastic heart shaped decoration.
NOW it is your turn. What blessing would you like to give to
Jennie? What gift would you like to give to Jennie? Remember in
drama anything is possible. Use your imagination. We have a drama
gift shop and we can shop there during the COVID-19 pandemic.
This gift shop has many departments.
Can you tell us a story that shows why Jennie is truly wonderful?
I want to thank Jennie for thinking about adding psychodrama
to your weekly schedule and not stopping until her co-counselor
Howie recommended me.

Before we close the session with another YouTube version of Happy
Birthday, Jennie takes the opportunity to address each and every person
in our Zoom Group and say something special to each one. This is her
spontaneous reaction to such a moving birthday experience.

Homework

Try to think of a birthday celebration in your life that was very special.

Zoom Session #6

May 27, 2020
   "We had such a wonderful birthday celebration last week.
   Tomorrow we celebrate the birthday of the giving of the Torah. *Sha-vuot*, (Pentecost), is a special holiday, as are all our Jewish holidays. When I say the word *Shavuot*, what do you think of? Raise your hand and we will unmute you". Celebrating in Jerusalem is especially exciting. In this

session, we actually are able to come close to the atmosphere we had created in our room at the center. The people are connecting. They are comfortable and they are communicating.

Here Is a Brief Summary

After reminding the members of our group of the birthday celebration from the week before, associations with the holiday come easily: dairy food, the Torah, learning. Learning Torah all night, eating cheesecake, wearing white, flowers. They actually mention all of the customs of this holiday and are able to connect to the holiday and to the replies of others. Their vernacular is from the old days and they enjoy hearing colloquial Yiddish words like *milchig* (dairy). The ritual of playing music and You-Tube at the beginning and end of our sessions is a stimulating challenge for me in my preparation and is a successful way of connecting them to the subject. I announce at the opening of the session that due to restrictions because of the COVID-19 situation, we will be unable to actually attend services at our local synagogues. Instead, the synagogue will come to our COVID-19 room! Yes, in drama anything can happen. I then ask Nancy to play the YouTube of the Hampton men's Choir singing every version of a very traditional prayer called *Adon Olam.* They enjoy this immensely and it transports them to the rituals of our holiday services. They sing along. I try to keep the YouTubes short. In many cases, I simply divide them so that they hear one half at the opening and the second half at the closing.

How many times in this book have I mentioned Moreno's expression "Trust the Process"? I use it in every session because it has proven to be so true. I decide to ask Nancy, our COVID-19 Zoom host, if she has an association for this holiday. I think it is important for the staff and the volunteers to be open and to participate. Nancy's association for this holiday is that it is her birthday. (Incidentally, this is my next subject, as their homework was to recall memories of birthdays.) Nancy does something amazing by sharing personal information with us. She tells us that fifteen years ago, on this holiday, she became a Jew. Despite it being a very personal story, Nancy describes the process in detail. Everyone is moved by this declaration and it becomes the perfect trigger for them to share personal stories of their birthdays with the group. I thank her for sharing this personal information and for trusting us. I explain that this is exactly what we are trying to do in this COVID-19 Zoom Group. I encourage the group to use this opportunity to tell one another things about ourselves that we want to share. Nancy has helped us build trust. Everyone is touched by her story and understands the benefits of sharing personal stories, not only in our sessions at the Melabev center but also here in our Zoom circle.

Moe tells us about the surprise 97th birthday party.

Bill shares how he organized a surprise birthday party for his wife's 60th birthday. We enjoy a few more examples of surprise parties.

Barbara remembers her sixth birthday. A few hours before the party, she was already dressed in a party dress, ready to welcome her friends. Unfortunately, her mother suddenly realized that she had never given out the invitations. They were still in her pocketbook. What should she do?! Barbara is very dramatic and articulate. Her mother was resourceful and went out to the street and found a bunch of children playing outside. She invited them all to come in and celebrate Barbara's birthday. I ask Barbara to give this birthday party story a name. Her apt response is, "A surprise birthday party!"

Moshe shares a photograph of his entire family – four generations. He shows it to us. What an opportunity! This was his most precious birthday present.

I ask the group if anyone wants to give Nancy a blessing for her birthday which will be coming up in a few days. They love to do this. They say meaningful things and wish her everything a person could ever want. The most moving is when Moe finds a sign from his 99th birthday and holds it up. It says HAPPY BIRTHDAY NAUGHTY 99. This is his way to express a wonderful wish of longevity with vitality.

More connections come from Miriam, who is an elderly volunteer, who has been attending all of our sessions and contributes by her enthusiastic and authentic participation. She shares the story of her husband's 90th birthday celebration. Because of COVID-19, they had to cancel the celebration but nevertheless, all of their children and grandchildren came to their building with balloons and good spirits. They all sang to him from the street. Another couple on our Zoom responds by saying, when they heard the singing, they went out onto their porch and joined in the celebration without knowing whose birthday they were celebrating. Yes, it certainly is possible to connect on the screen.

Zoom Session #7

June 3, 2020

Since the onslaught of COVID-19, home has taken on a new meaning for all of us. This session will focus on what home is for me.

Opening ritual: Hugging and connecting with our hands and arms.

Opening segment of music as a warm-up: "HOME SWEET HOME" YouTube performed by Erutan.

Our participants love to learn new facts. I google the song from a classic that they all recognize.

"Home Sweet Home" was written by American lyricist John Howard Payne and English composer Sir Henry Bishop for an opera that was first produced in London in 1823. The song became hugely popular throughout the United States and was a favorite of both Union and Confederate soldiers during the Civil War.

I recite the beautiful lyrics with sensitivity and a lot of expressions:

Lyrics

chorus:
Home! Home!
Sweet, sweet home!
There's no place like home
There's no place like home
verses:
'Mid pleasures and palaces
Though I may roam
Be it ever so humble
There's no place like home
A charm from the sky
Seems to hallow us there
Which seek thro' the world
Is ne'er met with elsewhere
To thee, I'll return
Overburdened with care
The heart's dearest solace
Will smile on me there
No more from that cottage
Again I will roam
Be it ever so humble
There's no place like home
I then proceed:

Today we are going to take advantage of the fact that we are all at our homes. Listen to this song and let it inspire you to connect to objects in YOUR HOME that will help tell us something about you – your life, your interests.

We all watch YouTube which shows nostalgic pictures of homes from years ago including sentimental objects in the home and outdoor scenes. The sweet magic of the music and the beautiful photos on the screen transport our audience to the homes and scenery of their childhood.

After we return to our gallery view, I can feel that they are ALL connected by this beautiful, heartwarming, virtual warm-up. I continue with my plans by adopting the theme of "There is no place like home." That's what Dorothy said in the Wizard of Oz.

I remind them of some of their responses two years ago when, after I had just seen a performance of the Wizard of Oz, and had asked them – What is home for each of you?

* "My family."
* "A place where I feel totally comfortable."
* "My own clean bathroom."
* "A place that is safe."

- "Israel is my home! I never felt at home in London."
- "This room."

I proceed to ask them, "Can you add to this?"

Barbara: "Home is where, when you get there, they have to let you in. Home is my parents' home where I grew up, my grandparents' home, where I spent a lot of time, and my home when I was married. They are all home in different ways – memories, different memories. They all came up when I listened to this song. Oh . . . and the home I live in today!"

The process continues. You can see on our Zoom screen that all of our participants are connected. No one is sleeping. Everyone is sitting close to the screen. The women on the staff and I can see their eyes roaming the screen. Everyone seems eager for more. We can all feel the energy. We can feel the memories evoking the need to tell, share and, hopefully, to show.

I continue my refrain, "What is home for you?"

Meir raises his hand. He continues with a disquieting story. He tells us that he had two childhood homes. These are his words:

> When I was six, my parents decided that I would not go to public school where we lived, in Denver. So, they shipped me away, to another home in New York, to live with my Bubbe (grandmother) my father's mother, of blessed memory. She was such a nice lady. For the next fifteen years I lived with her so that I could go to a yeshiva (a religious school with the emphasis on Torah learning) on the lower East Side.

I ask him the name of the yeshiva. When he replies "Rabbi Jacob Joseph" at least four or five of the participants clap or nod or smile in recognition of one of the oldest yeshivas in New York. They are definitely listening to his story. They are attuned. He continues, "I got to my parents' home in the summers and sometimes on holidays."

He has fond memories of both homes but there is a melancholy tone to his voice. He feels comfortable telling us this story filled with ambivalence. I actually ask him "Meir, you just told us a very emotional story. What are you feeling now?" He replies, "A longing. I still have it in my memory and in my heart. I have been with my wife wherever we have lived, for 62 years. That is home, wherever we are."

I continue: "Meir, when you think of the home you built with your wife, what emotion are you feeling?" He responds:

> Love, appreciation. The greatest feeling of home is to be here in Israel. We came in 1970 with all of our children, four boys and five girls. They are all here with their families. I am only sad that we have the COVID-19 and they can't visit us now.

I take this opportunity to ask everyone to look at all the boxes on the screen, at the Zoom Room we have created in order to point out to them that EVERYONE on the screen has made Israel their home. It was a choice. There are smiles in every box. Yes, they all have something in common.

Libby is very excited. Her aide speaks for her. She says:

> On behalf of Grand-mom Libby, home for us is a place where you can mingle with each other *good*; there's unity. If there is not unity, we cannot call it home; it is broken. I am in the home of the Goldman family; I call it home because I am happy with them.

(Her arm is around Libby who is smiling at her so lovingly. Libby gives her a hug.)

Geoffrey raises his hand and says with emotion, "Home is security for me and I can't go into details because I haven't got any details. I was two when my father was murdered by the Nazis." He is speaking fluently with no trouble expressing himself. This is an amazing accomplishment for him. He is totally coherent. He then adds, "I am glad this 'program' has given me the opportunity to say this." He is calm, composed and speaking independently. He is expressing something very close to his heart and the language is flowing with ease. This is a "moment" for the entire staff.

After I respond to Geoffrey I continue, "Who else wants to tell us what home is for them?" When no one raises their hand, I ask individuals. They always respond when asked directly. "Sarah, what is home for you?"

Susan:	Home is a place where my children grew up; I can see them every day and they are a joy to me.
Yehudit continues,	"Home is a comfortable place for my children."
Brian tells us	"I travelled a lot and lived in many places. Home was not just a place but home was always a special experience of 'Mama and Papa' ". He becomes agitated and very sad and distraught. Difficult memories are surfacing. I mirror him and say, "Brian, thinking of home is making you very sad. I am reaching my arms out to you to touch you. Can you feel it?" He replies, "Of course."
	I ask him to look around in his home today and think: "What is home for me right now?"
Brian replies:	"I've had so many homes in my life. Home has its own connotation."
	I repeat, "The word home is making you very sad."

He continues, "Maybe I am being harsh but life took home away from me. Place doesn't mean a damn to me. *Home was my life.* I'll never get over that." I respond empathically, "It is reminding you of a childhood that makes you very sad." "Absolutely! It destroys me." This is a recurring theme for him in our sessions.

Brian had a few childhood traumas that we have worked on a lot in our "before COVID-19" sessions through role reversals and short vignettes with his brothers, parents and son. I try to focus him on the loveliness of his life today. I feel that he is very agitated and emotionally flooded. I don't want him to break down here in the middle of a Zoom session. It is time to help him calm down and for me to focus on the rest of the group. It is indeed difficult to hold the participants on the screen but when I reach out with my two arms, I feel that I do touch him and reach him. I ask him if it is okay to turn to other participants. Holding his head, he nods giving his consent. I can sense his composure, or, perhaps, resignation, and decide that we can move on. This is not the right time or place to open this heavy subject again.

Hannah: "My home makes me very happy. It is comfortable, nice neighborhood, nice neighbors."

I respond that she brought us two important words – neighbors and comfortable.

Moe: "Home is the comfortable place you look forward to come back to after work."

Herbie: is not able to connect but he is listening intently. I ask his wife to ask him what home is for him. He ends up saying simply, "Home is sweet."

When I turn to **Deena,** she responds: My family was very big, seven children. I am thinking of my father – his singing. Home is listening to my father singing.

I interject, "Yes, home is family music. The songs we sang together." I thank her for that wonderful contribution. I would like to let them share songs from their homes. Maybe we can do that in a different session.

As you can see, it is alright for me to turn to them and ask if and when they do not volunteer. These are people who are not used to expressing such delicate, intimate information.

I proceed with my plan.

"Look around at your home today. Can you find an object in your home that will help tell us something about you, your life or your interests?"

Again, there is zero response so I continue by showing them my favorite coffee mug and explaining how home is where I like to sit down and have a cup of coffee with someone. I love inviting people in my life to come over for a cup of coffee since I do not like coffee shops.

I prepared the staff to feel free to volunteer to answer and act as a trigger, when the group is slow in responding. This always worked before COVID-19.

Jennie opens up the subject and is the trigger. She shows us a wall filled with photos. I ask the group to raise their hands if they have photos around them. Almost everyone raises their hand and proceeds to show us intimate collages of their lives. They are able to show and share – not imaginary but real photos. We can feel the excitement.

Barbara is reminded of the windup Victrola thanks to Devora's mention of music. I comment, "I was expecting you to bring objects from today, but the nostalgic music from the YouTube is definitely transporting all of us to the past."

All through the session, I notice **Herbie** getting up and looking for something. This is not easy for his wife, Bea. In this case, Zoom does not let us help him become more focused and less overwrought. But he is nonetheless, engaged. He is much more connected when his wife sits with him rather than his aide.

We encounter many objects from their homes displayed with pride and a lot of expressions. We get to see a bottle of wine that was saved from Mike's 51st wedding anniversary celebration, a whiskey glass that tells us of Herbie's habit of drinking a *glozzele shnappes* – a shot of whiskey, when he came home from work each day, Bernard's gold coin from Ethiopia and, of course, many photos that tell many stories and lets us see their families.

We finally hear from **Ed**. For him, home is a quiet place. I thank him profusely for this important contribution. Yes, home is where we can find our quiet peaceful place.

Herbie finds what is home for him when we also meet **Herbie** and Bea's cat, Moochie. I ask all those who ever had a pet to raise their hands. It is important to use every opportunity to encourage participation. It keeps the participants alert and helps them feel a social cohesion even on the screen.

We end with an instrumental version of the song, Home Sweet Home.

Before ending the session, we finally succeed in unmuting the one person we had not heard from, **Mendy**. He closes our session by saying that home is a sanctuary for him. Moreover, he knows we have not given up on him. What he has to say is important.

This session was indeed very moving. The participants were very present and involved. For the first time in Zoom land, I did not have to work hard. There was a comfortable flow.

Actually, my choice of YouTube for the opening of the session was a perfect trigger. The photos and the quality of the sweet singing transported the people almost magically to the homes of their childhood and hence to themselves. Finding an object from their home that could tell us something about them created an atmosphere that was invigorating, intimate and inviting. Somehow it also turned into *reminiscence therapy* since most of the associations and objects were from their past.

By the end of the session, EVERYONE had spoken and everyone was cherishing the words of their friends. Throughout the session, I was conducting but Nancy and Jennie were noticing all the nuances of the people in their groups. Their devotion is always a great contribution to the success of the meeting and they notice everything.

I thank the participants for sharing their homes and memories with us. I am sure they are happy for the opportunity and are waiting for more.

This session is written up by Nancy, Chariklia and myself in: Brown, N., Cedar, T., Tziraki, C. (2022). Psychodrama with persons with dementia on Zoom: Proof of concept. *Dementia: The International Journal of Social Research and Practice.*

Zoom Session # 8

July 24, 2020

Celebrating a 100th birthday on Zoom.

How often does one get to celebrate a 100th birthday on Zoom? This celebration was a special first time for all of us, and I'm writing about it in the past tense because it's all about the past. The staff and six hand-picked guests from our group all recited the *Shehechiyanu*, the prayer which is said when one is doing or experiencing something from which one derives pleasure or benefit for the first time. We all said it together. This was not planned. It was a spontaneous emotional outpouring of gratitude for the opportunity to experience this momentous occasion together and on Zoom, no less.

Yes, our Moe, who was "the oldest tree in the forest" (see opening section, The Forest), had reached 100. It is not often that one is given the privilege of working with a person who, it is certain, never said an unkind word to anyone.

What a pleasure it was to gather together a small group of people who knew Moe well and wanted to pay tribute to him and his life. I was asked to plan something that would take no longer than ten minutes. The entire Zoom would be short as Moe's attention span is short. He also has trouble staying awake. I will share my thought process in planning my part in this major celebration. Ten minutes is much more difficult than a half-hour. Especially for me!!

I thought about the significance of the number 100. I then googled what happened 100 years ago. Who was born in 1920? What began in 1920? What was life like in those days? It was all very intriguing. I then thought about our sweet, kind-hearted humorous Moe.

After opening, I reminded him and the other participants (reminders are always useful with this population) of many of his responses in our sessions. Moe's comments have always been sharp and sweet.

Fortunately, Howie, our music man, was the official host of this celebration. I had suggested that he open with a song and he did. He actually had us all join him in the singing of a very melodic catchy version of the words to the blessing of *Shehechiyanu.*

For my drama activity, I ask the participants, "If we were to write a book or make a film about Moe's life, what would be the title?" This is a sure way to summarize one hundred years? I cannot emphasize this enough! Naming or giving a title helps our participants focus on the essence of a subject. Their replies were indeed a perfect encapsulation of Moe's essence. Moe is not in a state of mind where he can answer but **Barbara** steps right in with a great title, "Keep Moving Forward and Onward". **Harvey** raises his hand and offers the title: "A Time Well Spent".

I try for more ideas and ask **Brian** who is having trouble keeping his head up. This celebration is making him feel old and tired. He is 93. But he says, "Anything is inadequate."

I rephrase in order to get a response from Moe. "What would be a good name for these 100 years? Moe, you've seen everything. What are the things you have seen?" Sometimes Moe acts his age and does not respond. He seems lost. One of our volunteers pitches in, "The bravery of all the people who left everything to move to Israel." He nods his head in agreement.

I focus in on Moe.

> Moe, you once shared with us how you fell in love with your wife. You told us that you first saw her on the stage in an elementary school assembly. You told us that usually men don't like girls with glasses but you definitely liked her.

This warms him up and he proceeds to tell us about their first kiss. Our party participants are enjoying celebrating their dear friend's life. They smile at every word.

He continues to express himself. He is now articulate and full of majestic yet simple eloquence.

> I didn't make a lot of money but I accomplished a lot with my family. I am not sorry about anything in my life. To be sorry means a life wasted. I did a lot. I did not waste my time. I did volunteer work. I learned this from years of watching my mother do *schnorring* – a Yiddish word for collecting money for good causes.

Moe enjoys using the language of the old world. He continues, "I wish I could say on my 100th birthday that I am more alert. My friends are ALL younger than me! An achievement I am proud of is that my daughter's friends are glad that I am still around."

All of his statements are so simple, honest and pure. He receives a compliment, "You are so sharp and with it." And he is, some of the time.

I then list a few things that happened 100 years ago. Band-aids were invented. Good Humor ice-cream started in 1920. Many famous people were born.

- Actors Walter Matthau, Tony Randall, Mickey Rooney
- "Star Trek" actors DeForest Kelley and James Doohan
- Scientist Isaac Asimov
- Writers Ray Bradbury, Mario Puzo ("The Godfather")
- Musician Charlie Parker
- Actress Shelley Winters
- Newsman David Brinkley
- Newswoman Hannah Thomas
- Violinist Isaac Stern
- Psychologist Timothy Leary
- Jazz musician Dave Brubeck

I summarize, "They are no longer with us, but Moe, you are still here." I would like to sum up what was said in this short session. It is important for the participants to hear their name and to repeat what they have just said. Saying names keeps the group members awake and alert.

> Harvey, you said that these 100 years of Moe's life was a time well spent and Barbara you said that Moe's 100 years could be called moving onward and forward. Moe your 100 years was a time well spent by moving on and moving forward with good humor and Moe you put a band-aid on anyone who needed it to make them better.

Everyone, on our screen, is thrilled to participate in this unique celebration of life. I would like to give this session the title "A Love Story".

Summary of Practical Applications

- People with dementia are capable of connecting and participating actively in group work online. Despite the challenges of technology, this can actually be an easier kind of exposure.
- Using sound and movement keeps the participants, on the screen, alert and involved.
- Using share-screen can be useful for stimulation, background, music, videos, and so on.
- It *is* possible to build a circle of trust on the screen by encouraging the participants to look at all the squares and interact.
- Spectrograms and other forms of sociometry can be revised for interaction on the screen by showing from 0 to 10 with your hands.
- Sharing the home environment presents the leader with new opportunities for connection and provides us with another perspective to the lives of our group members.

- The intimacy of meeting from everyone's home allows new creative ways of "*touching*" one another.
- Through the Zoom sessions, we learned that this population, despite cognitive limitations, can be engaged, can communicate naturally and can expand.
- Zoom sessions should be well planned but the leader's spontaneity is the most essential component for true success.

Creating a New Group Between Lockdowns

The Melabev Center reopened in the summer of 2020 during one of the intervals of COVID-19, and as a result, Zoom sessions ceased. The actual functioning and organization at the center became very different, and initially, because of my age, I did not return to work there. I was waiting for the healthy, unmasked world before COVID-19. Our Zoom sessions became an experiment in the making. I learned to create an atmosphere of trust, safety, expression, connection and belonging through action on the screen. The fact that these sessions worked so well proves to what extent our participants are hungry for social cohesion and validation via group work – even on a screen.

When it became safe due to the successful vaccination campaign in Israel in spring 2021, I was asked to return and build a new group. There were many adjustments that I had to make in my therapeutic work at Melabev. Our population, which had been living with many unknowns, had also endured fifteen months with anxiety, loneliness, boredom and lethargy. In many ways, they were post-trauma from the COVID-19 pandemic.

Many people did not return to the center. Those who did return were at a lower level in their physical and cognitive functioning and I had to integrate them with new members to create and build a new cohesive group. I reread PART II of this book, and worked on improving my method. I am going to share what I learned from the first group and which techniques I used to help create a new safe circle of trust. My previous experience with this population was invaluable but the most significant tools were flexibility, spontaneity and creating a comfortable atmosphere filled with humor, openness and honesty. Fortunately, my tools helped people connect to me, to psychodrama, to one another and to themselves. They could feel validated. I did as many *doubles* as possible and used a sociometric spectrogram by having the group raise their hands from 0 to 10 in order to identify with what was said by others. Throwing the pillow to someone else in the group was an activity that they loved. When I had them throw the pillow to the person whose name comes next alphabetically, in order to help them recognize others in the group by their name, one man said, "I don't know who she is!" I replied, "Now you will" and he understood and agreed. When a new member, aged 96, threw the pillow, I crowned her as the oldest basketball player in the world. She was wary of staying at the center at her introductory session and now, she did not want to leave.

> . . . the most significant tools were flexibility, spontaneity and creating a comfortable atmosphere filled with humor, openness and honesty.

In order to explain what we would be doing together, in these psychodrama sessions, I created a ritual. In this ceremony that opened each session, I let my animal puppets be my assistants. This is a form of projection and *concretizing*. For example, the peacock tells them that I want to help them spread their wings and realize their potential as I make the puppet spread its wings aesthetically. The parrot sends the message that here in our psychodrama sessions, we open our mouths, express our feelings and tell our story. The zebra validates that it is okay to feel different – from what we were in the past and from the people in our lives today. The owl reminds them that their life-long experiences have given them wisdom. The turtle helps them accept their slower pace and their need for protection. The butterfly advises them to free themselves from anxiety, doubt, frustration, bitterness and seek out the beauty in nature. They eventually met many more puppets with important messages. This was also a way to acquaint them slowly with my array of puppets so that I would be able to conduct later sessions using them. (See PART III Projection with Puppets.)

With this new group, I would walk in and meet a new member who had no idea what psychodrama was. Also, many of the original participants could not even remember who I was. This opening ritual and the physical setup of sitting in the circle with no tables helped them all connect to the weekly psychodrama session. As soon as I saw that something was too abstract and difficult for them, I would make the appropriate adjustment. My main goal was to achieve trust in themselves, one another, the method, and of course myself, as the facilitator. I knew that trust was being built when a first-time participant said to me from her seat at the lunch table:

> I need to talk to you privately . . . actually, I can tell you right here in front of these other women! I am having a hard time. I feel guilty because I am so dependent on my children now that I have Alzheimer's and can't function.

The other women at her table immediately identified with what she said validated her. I thanked her for bringing up a subject that is so important to everyone in the group and said that I would work on it in our next session.

Actually, I could write another chapter on how my experiences these past six years contributed to starting all over with a new group and a new *me*. In this successive beginning, I started out with the hope that was based on our journey together from 2015 to the present. Writing this handbook has helped me develop and deepen my approach to using psychodrama with this special population. I still arrive at each session and each challenge with the hope that there will be a creation or a discovery or an *action insight* that will give validation to the strengths, needs and uniqueness of each person in our circle and the value of our group work. This attitude is what I have been trying to project onto this group. I have been striving to reinforce their sense of *twinship*, belonging and allowing our process to heal their sense of isolation and loneliness, so intensified by the COVID-19 pandemic. At the same time, I was striving to give the individuals in the Group an identity that fills them with dignity. Here an inspirational quote from Rabbi Dr. Jonathan Sacks is very apt: "I prefer the word hope to optimism. Optimism is the belief that things will get better; hope is the belief that *together* we can make things better" (Sacks, 2019, Covenant and Conversation: Genesis p. 256).

Summary of Practical Applications

- It is possible to create a new group that is made up of people from the original group and new members.
- When building a new group, it is wise to learn from our mistakes as well as our achievements.
- Using puppets to deliver a message in the opening ritual, is an invitation to the participants to join in.

Part VIII

Beyond the Process

Sharing My Thoughts

In Hebrew the word *hazara* means going back to the past and also means rehearsal for something in the future. This is precisely what transpired in our psychodrama sessions. The participants were able to retrieve memories from the past, share them and ultimately learn about themselves and gain strengths and new insights into their present situation. These memories facilitated an improved self-image with more self-confidence and positive energy to move on into their future.

Our participants experienced "holding" in a safe environment. This form of therapy, through drama, definitely had a healing and cathartic effect on these elderly people who were coping with so many difficulties. I learned a lot about all the members of the group and gained wisdom about life from each and every one of them. They are open and honest and come to our sessions with hope.

I am so much more sensitive to the challenges facing caregivers to this population. I have also learned a lot about myself, through the participants, because it is impossible not to gain deep awareness from psychodrama. Thank you, Moreno, for inspiring me to trust the process!

Sharing From Members of Our Staff

There are populations where we need to rely on others in order to be most effective. At Melabev, I learned not to be a soloist, and instead to rely on the staff and work with others. Actually, all group leaders experience a form of loneliness when they direct an independent therapy group. This experience of working with a staff of professionals and volunteers was enriching, supportive and helped me grow. All the group leaders; Howie, Gila, Frances were perfect partners in our psychodrama sessions. They all participated and contributed spontaneously, eagerly and devotedly. There were actually times when Jennie, the leader in charge of the group, would whisper essential information while I was in the throes of an enactment so that I would not go too far

DOI: 10.4324/9781003321705-8

with a specific participant. The *twinship* between us was always palpable and beneficial.

Michal, our talented volunteer, was our auxiliary ego whenever necessary. Her sharing from the role, after an enactment, became a source of direct validation and empathic encouragement for our participants.

When Chariklia, this center's medical consultant, sat in on a session, she would sum up with an empowering comment. We would meet after the session and she would share her observations with me and translate them into the professional language that helped me grow in this endeavor. Her comments told me that people came alive in the psychodrama sessions, and helped me understand that from a medical point of view, it was their best medicine.

When all of us met after our Zoom sessions during the closure due to the pandemic and we shared our observations, I felt validated and motivated by the sharing and feedback of the other members of the staff. They were always so excited by the *action* and interaction . . . on a screen.

There were many people on the staff who contributed their skills and sensitivities to our sessions. I asked a few to share their experience of sitting in our circle to show you how essential they were for our participants and for me in our process.

Here is what Jennie wrote:

> **Jennie:** Our Center was opening up an additional day for our group, the Challenge Group. We would now be available to our group's clients five days a week. The Director of the Center asked me if there was anything in particular I would like to incorporate in this new day's program.
>
> I am a pretty spontaneous person and replied immediately, "Yes, inner work!" I wanted something that would enable the clients to access and talk about their inner world. No program was relating to their feelings about all they are going through in relation to independence, faltering memory, medical situation, family members and their relationships with them.
>
> All our programs in Melabev are centered around creating a cheerful atmosphere. Any opportunity for a party was always welcome, be it a birth of a grandchild or great-grandchild, a birthday or any family celebration. However, I felt there was an additional element we could explore within our Challenge Group population.
>
> The reason someone is assigned to our Group is because these are people who are still in the early stages of Alzheimer's who still retain varying higher levels of ability and desire for social interaction. Coming from a background in social work, I felt it was very important to maximize their verbal skills, to give them a chance to talk about their feelings, their worries and the concerns about their

current lives. I did not have a picture of how this would be achieved but after meeting Tzippi and working together for a few weeks, I had a good feeling that together we would be able to Trust the Process to achieve these goals.

The group she came into was already a well-established group of people of whom many recognized and remembered each other from week to week. Not everyone comes every day. Their response to Tzippi was warm and willing to give this woman, with her "Bag of Schmattes" a chance.

The members of the Group were asked to suggest subjects they would like to work on. The topics sounded wide and varied but really boiled down to a few main points. "I am not being heard." "I have lost my voice in my family." As the Group became more familiar with this interesting technique, their trust grew. Sometimes our session would take off fast. I felt very protective of each member of the group and would sometimes have to catch her mid-sentence to be sure her question or comment to someone was within the bounds of their ability to cope.

As one person's drama would be unfolding the whole group would remain silent, focused on the dynamics being played out. There was always an atmosphere of unity and respect. Everyone knew that what was happening in the room was important. This was a unique and special time for the *protagonists* to be open and honest because they were being "heard".

Since the staff was definitely an integral part of the session and not an audience it facilitated opportunities to use information that only I was aware of, in order to trigger expressions that might help meet their specific needs. The responses that these sessions evoked provided important information about deep conflicts, inner strengths, capabilities and needs that could be addressed at the center.

As the months went by, this became the session that everybody waited for. This had become a safe place for them to share their most private, and sometimes not so "pretty" feelings. They felt empowered, (even if for some, it only lasted a short time). They were reminded of their accomplishments in their lives. Some of these people were leaders in their fields, brilliant innovators and ingenious creators. They regained their pride.

For me personally, and as the Group's leader, these sessions have given me a deep sense of satisfaction. Tzippi and her expert use of psychodrama techniques have proven to be a most effective and enhancing tool to help our clients. These people, whose skills in communication are declining and whose self-esteem is ebbing away partly because of a lack of meaningful involvement, have benefited immensely. During our group time, they sat up straighter, listened eagerly and participated enthusiastically. There was laughter and sometimes tears and a deep sense of belonging and achievement.

Michal volunteered in our group with love, devotion and a deep sense of responsibility. We had met in a small gift shop and started talking. When I told her what I do, she exclaimed, "I am studying psychodrama, could I please come to one of your groups to observe how you work with them?" My instant reply was, "I don't believe it is correct or ethical to have an audience in a psychodrama session." Then I suggested to Michal to come to our center and volunteer in our group. This way she could be an official member of our staff. "Trust the Process" very quickly, Michal became our professional auxiliary ego in our vignettes, role reversals and enactments. She was a natural at this and a gift for all of us.

Here is what Michal wrote:

> Michal: My role as an auxiliary ego in psychodramas with the Challenge Group at the Melabev Center took me some time to do well. It was necessary to get to *know and feel* the individuals, to know how they felt in their souls. Playing the role of someone they loved like their wife or a son of theirs in their real lives required them to have a high level of trust in me.
>
> This trust was something that developed over time in our psychodrama meetings. For a person to allow me to hug them after playing the role of their wife was a warm highlight for me. I was moved to do it because I had grown to deeply care about and feel very close to the individuals in our group. Aside from thoroughly enjoying my role with this group, I was amazed at the depths we were able to reach in our people's worlds. We were able to offer them different options that did not present themselves in the experiences of their actual lives.
>
> Another aspect of this role for me was my thorough enjoyment and the use of creativity that I tapped into when playing the diverse roles that arose so spontaneously. I experienced such satisfaction from playing these meaningful roles and helping our people reach an empathic understanding of situations in their relationships.
>
> A huge side benefit was having the opportunity to gain insight into and connecting with my own internal emotional issues.

The many social work students who were doing their practicum at Melabev over these years loved seeing and witnessing how attentive and responsive our group members were at these psychodrama sessions. I insisted that they also participate. After each session, they shared their excitement at seeing how psychodrama could draw on the imagination, feelings, sense of humor and level of innate intelligence of each patient.

Noah, one of the student social workers, who now works at Melabev, wrote about his experience:

> I quickly learned that the classic therapeutic experience wasn't used with individuals with dementia because it was too challenging due to memory impairment. However, as my work continued, therapy took on a whole new meaning. In this group, I witnessed and learned that individuals with dementia do not only benefit from the psycho-drama therapeutic process and express and share insight into their personal experience, but they also support one another in a way that no one else can.

Learning From the Process

In PART I of this book, I introduced you to a sampling of the people who have participated in our sessions since September 2015 until the COVID-19 pandemic in March 2020 in order to "show|" you the character and energy of our Group and share my first impressions. This was my way of inviting you to sit in our circle. I did not know too much about the families, the illnesses, strengths and weaknesses of these people. Now that you have witnessed our interaction, I want to share what I learned from our process together. In order to protect their privacy, the individual names have been changed, and collective information will be shared.

Self-Image

The members of this group were genuinely honest about themselves and their limitations, full of self-criticism and guilt about the burden they have become for their spouse and offspring.

They felt shame and were critical of themselves.

There was remorse and regret that needed to be expressed and processed.

The process encouraged transparency. The leader and the staff were open and transparent when appropriate. This certainly invited comfortable disclosure from the participants.

They needed to be reminded of their incredible accomplishments as scholars in the academic world, engineers, museum curators, authors, physicians, nurses, survivors, heads of departments and successful businessmen.

They needed validation and hope in every aspect of their lives. Not being able to retrieve essential information can cause a total shutdown. On the other hand, tiny triggers can activate their memory.

In many cases, their hours at Melabev were the happiest parts of their weekly routines.

Social Image

The members of our Group were alone in their inner experiences and had a deep sense of loneliness. They needed social cohesion and a sense of belonging.

They needed exercises and techniques such as role reversals to expand their empathy to other people in their lives. Close identification with the others in the group led to compassion and empathy for one another. The intimacy from the psychodramatic enactments instilled them with confidence and vitality.

Pressure on current family relationships due to their illnesses weighed heavily upon them.

Our work uncovered unfinished business needing to receive closure.

People who have been highly intelligent, cultured, well-read and passionate remain all these when they are stricken with dementia. They have a sense of humor and are interested in learning and advancing and are sociable human beings. More than anything else, these people needed and received validation from one another.

Medical Aspects

Alzheimer's disease and other forms of dementia do not exclude other medical conditions that need to be addressed.

Parkinson's disease can affect cognition, language and memory.

Lewy Body Disease causes confusion, hallucinations and impairs functioning. BUT there are times when those suffering from it surprise themselves and everyone around them and are coherent. It is essential to never give up and to stimulate as often as possible.

Cognition and functioning of the elderly are influenced by medication and vary according to the amount of sleep they are getting, their diet, the amount of exercise they take and the degree of tension in their lives.

Dementia defies dignity. The antidote is respect, attention, interaction and, of course, validation.

High-functioning Alzheimer patients CAN remember when properly stimulated.

Social interaction stimulates cognition and genuine communication is possible.

Memory is easily retrieved when triggered by subjects that are close to their hearts.

People with Alzheimer's disease and other forms of dementia still have values, principles, determination and simple needs.

There are many ripple effects to these conditions. Spouses and offspring need and want to hear good things about their loved ones. This is both a terrible and a frightening loss for them. They also need to feel appreciated and included in the process. Assistance and support are essential to the caretakers' constant need to help the patient cope with his or her daily existence.

More About the Participants From the Original Group and the Post-COVID-19 Group

In the opening section of this book I shared my first impressions of various members of this group at the beginning of our process. My purpose was to introduce the dynamic makeup of this group. I quickly learned that in order to achieve therapeutic results, I would have to adapt many of my methods to the diverse levels of basic functioning in this group. Some of the members also suffered from emotional conditions such as bipolar disorder, paranoia and depression. In doing so, the people in our circle became my teachers. On the one hand, they surprised me with their intelligence and insightful comments and responses. On the other hand, their honesty about their limitations and frustrations helped me adapt to each person's innate needs. One of the most poignant comments was made to me by Joyce, a new participant in our post-COVID-19 group, after her second session with us, "I love the way you see each and every one of us and how what you do helps each of us see ourselves!" I know that these psychodramatic techniques help people feel seen, recognized, heard and, of course, validated.

> "I love the way you see each and every one of us and how what you do helps each of us see ourselves!"

To emphasize this point, I would like to share a sweet story. Once, at a wedding, the young waitress at our table looked at me and said, "You're Tzippi Cedar! Don't you remember me? You did psychodrama with our class in the seventh grade!" Obviously, I did not remember her as I have worked with hundreds of people each year. But my response helped this 22-year-old understand her excitement at seeing me after all these years. I replied, after asking her name and age:

> What a compliment! I am so glad you feel this way because that shows me that what we did in all of those sessions helped you connect to yourself and YOU remember yourself and how you felt and what you learned in those sessions.

Getting back to the new post-COVID-19 group, I will share some basic background information on more members in our original group and others who joined up later on in this process and the effects of psychodrama on how they presented in our experiential sessions. (This explains the unevenness in these brief descriptions.) Not only did I learn about the feelings, needs and yes, even the passions of each person, but they each learned to appreciate themselves and one another through this interactive expressive therapy.

The new members who were recently admitted to the Melabev program are marked here by PC (post Covid). Others were not new to Melabev but had not been in our Tuesday morning group, and I had met them via our Zoom sessions during COVID-19. Others joined our initial group midway through our process.

Daniel: 84 years (PC) – had worked very successfully in the medical profession. After several strokes which caused blockage in his brain, he had vascular dementia. He had no memory of anything but was able to participate in the here and now of our sessions as if everything was fine. His *grandiosity* came from giving us short concerts on a trumpet he brought into the sessions. He remembered all his music. His self-confidence came from his positive upbeat attitude towards life and a very supportive family. He was a good listener and an active responder with a remarkably positive disposition.

Edward: 86 years (PC) – was a lawyer. He is suffering from functional deterioration. He was at first threatened by psychodrama but he realized how safe and soothing it was for him after he shared a personal life tragedy and did not feel exposed or uncomfortable. Then his attitude changed.

Jeanette: 80 years (PC) – was a lawyer. She is happily married and is in a wheelchair with severe damage from a stroke. She has a lot of thoughts to share but is deterred by the slur in her speech. Her demeanor is cheerful. She feels loved and held and has incredible dignity.

Joyce: 80 years (PC) – was a law editor. She is physically independent despite her severe diabetes. She comes to Melabev because she needs the company and the stimulation to keep her busy. Her husband is no longer capable of filling these needs as he is very ill and limited.

Libby: 90 years – has suffered a series of minor strokes plus one significant stroke. She had trouble finding words to express herself but managed to let us know how she was feeling. She repeatedly expressed her values as a proud family person who appreciates the honesty, safety and trust in our psychodrama group. My *doubles* for her made her sit up taller as she felt listened to and understood.

Manny: 70 years – had been a successful engineer. His difficult home situation and dementia resulting from a stroke made him very needy at Melabev. He responded appropriately when I approached him but he never initiated. On the other hand, he was an active listener. Although his responses were not dynamic, they were always consistent and sometimes surprisingly expressive and meaningful. In our sessions, he did not give up on himself and maintained his dignity.

Mitch: 85 years – had been a successful physician. He lives with his daughter's family and uses his superb sense of humor to cope with his advancing dementia and dependence.

Pearl: 78 years (PC) – was a physical and occupational therapist. Her functioning has seriously abated and she needs activities and stimulation. Meeting the other group members in our session convinced her to try out Melabev twice a week. She is highly functional and identified with many members of our circle.

Penny: 95 years (PC) – after a serious fall which led to limited physical activities, her cognition deteriorated. At first, she could not remember names. She had been an English teacher and a true scrabble champion. Whereas her demeanor was passive and sad, whenever she was approached by me in our psychodrama interactive sessions, her responses were witty, humorous and filled with vitality. According to the staff members, it was like a miracle.

Samantha: 85 years (PC) – has a Ph.D. in Literature. She taught English at a University and authored a book about the Holocaust. Being so fragile and dependent on her children because of her dementia is a new and disheartening issue for her.

Simon: 75 years – had been a family physician who suffers from dementia and depression. When he first came, he never initiated anything and kept his head down, projecting a depressive state and avoiding eye contact. All of this changed when a hospital treatment for severe back pain brought about a noticeable improvement in his ability to communicate. He actually has a terrific sense of humor. In our post-COVID-19 Wednesday morning group, he was able to connect to others and enjoy their reactions and respond with a new vitality.

Summary of Practical Applications

- When working with a population that is so challenged physically, mentally and emotionally, it is advisable to not work alone.
- Staff members should sit in the circle and contribute to the sessions through active participation, being auxiliary egos, sharing and taking care of specific needs (walking, drinks, bathroom breaks).

- Members of the staff spend many hours with the participants and have valuable information to share and their perspective is enlightening.
- After a six-year process, we discover.
- We learn a lot about the method, its strengths and weaknesses.
- We learn about the people we work with because the method paves a path into their inner worlds.
- We discover and become able to embrace so much about ourselves: our resilience, our vulnerability, our creativity and our commitment to helping others cope and continue.
- Trusting the Process of using Psychodrama with this population is an especially fulfilling experience.

Appendix

Further Illustrations

Introduction

Up till now, I have been writing about the group process over the past years. In this part of the Appendix, I want to add a section with a condensed elaboration on many of the subjects that were listed in order to give to you, the reader, more options that evoke response from this specifically challenged population and help people in all groups overcome loneliness. Some sessions are simply outlined. In others, I bring a sampling of responses. Others are described in detail whenever I feel the particular responses are significant. Reading and witnessing the genuine words and spontaneous responses in each of the following narratives are definitely a gift.

Just a quick reminder, I have been leading a psychodrama group with amazing people between the ages of 59 and 96, Tuesday mornings, at the Melabev day-care facility in Jerusalem. The participants in this particular group are high-functioning Alzheimer patients or are suffering from some cognitive decline caused by other illnesses or old age. And again, and again they have shown me that one CAN do psychodrama with Alzheimer patients!!!

At our sessions, I bring subjects that deal with the challenges of their daily life, coping with the changes in their physical and cognitive capabilities and accepting these changes with dignity and self-pride. As you become familiar with the range of subjects that I have brought here, I would like you to consider what your responses would be in all of these sessions. What does this do to you? When you think about it, do you gain new insights? Does it empower you? Do you think of things you have never really thought about? How does this journey inwards make you feel? From my experience, this could result in a more empathic connection to this population and to yourself.

The Melabev Day Care Facility in Jerusalem is a happy place for the right reasons. There is so much caring, sharing, creativity and genuine expression. The following sampling will open the door to our room so that you can peek in, see and amplify what went on in our sessions.

Elaboration of Sessions

The following are a selection of highlights from many sessions:

I Feel Old When . . .

Me – (As a warm-up trigger) I feel old when I feel pain.
Daisy – When I am tired and I can't remember things.
Miriam – (volunteer) When I look in the mirror.
Barbara – I feel old when I can't do things I used to do. I don't look in the mirror.
Martin – Why are we discussing being old?
Barbara – (jokingly) Why are you rubbing it in that we are old?
Deena – I feel old when I feel like people are taking advantage of me.
Michal – (volunteer) I feel old when I am climbing stairs.

I continue to build:
What do you do to feel young?
Following are a few samples:

Lila – By continuing to use my brain. By going out and going to classes.
Martin – When I go out to have a good time.
Barbara – Getting out of bed every morning to come to Melabev.

"No Place Like Home"

After seeing a production of "The Wizard of Oz" we talked about the show, recalled and sang some of the songs. This led to the famous quote from the show and the movie: *There is no place like home.* I asked our participants what HOME meant for them.
Here are a few of their responses:

- "My family."
- "A place where I feel totally comfortable."
- "My own clean bathroom."
- "A place that is safe."
- "Israel is my home! I never felt at home in London."

"This room."
And many more . . .

The Walker, Friendship

I was away for a week. I always return from a trip abroad with a bag of Hershey's Kisses. But . . . I forgot to bring them to the session. We have a good laugh and an even better deep connection. This is further proof that they are not alone with their issues. Yes, I also forget things. It is not comfortable and they experience my embarrassment. They share an empathic experience with me. I had forgotten the chocolates but I did not forget to bring my walker which I still needed for my broken leg.

We then use my walker as a concrete tool in this psychodrama session. I put it in the center of the circle and let them tell the walker whatever they want. They are now sharing another empathic experience with me. I know how it feels to need a walker, a wheelchair and a cane after I broke my leg on a bicycle trip.

Some of their comments addressed to the walker are:

Lila – I hope I won't need you.
Monica – I'm thankful you are here when I need you.
Daisy – You make me feel old.
Barbara – I wish you had a seat . . . and a motor.
Me – You help me stand up straight and keep my balance.
Martin – Why would someone your age go biking?! (He has been sleeping a lot in our sessions because of a new medication. This subject and my personal story have kept him awake and involved) He even gets a double from our amazing volunteer Michal, *"I worry about you Tzippi"*, which Martin proudly confirms.

Back to the session, I had carefully planned what I was going to do with them, after this warm-up but, other issues have come up. There are two new women in the group. Both are feeling very anxious. The situation about the chocolate Hershey's Kisses when I confessed that I can also forget, helped them feel more relaxed. I then spontaneously ask a few participants to introduce themselves with an adjective so that the new members could somehow feel more comfortable in the circle. This takes a few minutes. We actually hear a few new adjectives to add to our list: inquisitive, schlepping, intelligent, honest, fantastic! (This woman was obviously on medication. She is usually very grouchy and difficult. Today she was high!). The two new women are now ready to participate. One describes herself as anxious. The second one says she is everlasting, persistent. . . . She is having trouble finding the exact description. We work through a few doubles to understand that she means . . . determined. The two women are pleased with their responses. They feel more relaxed in our circle.

I am ready to start the session that I had planned. I even prepared the group for the innovative way I am going to do some sociometric exercises with all kinds of criteria but then Martin would like to ask a question in the midst of what I am doing. He actually tells me, "The only reason I came today was for this session." Of course, I answer in the affirmative and leave my plans for another session. I am glad that he feels comfortable to share an issue with the group. He asks, "What do we do when a friend is not nice . . . anymore?" Looks like he came today to try and find a solution to what was deeply troubling him. Yes, this is a therapy group! I spontaneously pull out a chair and place it in front of him.

I ask Martin, "What do you want to tell your friend?"

"We used to do things together. You liked going places with me. Now you are avoiding me. You don't spend any time with me and you hardly even talk to me."

By using the psychodramatic tool of the empty chair, we learn what is causing Martin's agitation. I let other people in the group talk to the imaginary friend in the chair so that Martin can feel less exposed and vulnerable.

I proceed with the question, "What do we do when a friend is not nice?" My instruction is, "Imagine your friend is in this chair. Now you can complain to this person about something that this person has done to hurt you." In order to get them started, I open with obvious genuine pain and I say to my imaginary friend in the empty chair, "Why didn't you invite me to your celebration? You invited all of our crowd. Why did you leave us out?" This warms them up and they continue.

Barbara – "Why don't you mind your own business?"
Adrienne – "Keep on calling, please!"
Daisy – "Why don't you accept me?"
Ruth – "You are sh-t!"
Benjy – "I'd like to tell my wife to get a hearing aid."
And then it comes . . . the truth . . . expressed with so much pain.
Martin – "We've been married for many years. We don't go out together anymore. You don't take me with you. I want to be closer."

He is talking to his second wife. His first wife, of many wonderful years together, passed away and he remarried. His second marriage was a good marriage until his situation deteriorated. He feels safe now to share his frustration and disappointment. That is enough for now. Opening this up to a vignette would be too much for him. Right now, he needs to express his disappointment and get validation for his frustration.

I then continue, "Let's try to think of what kind of friends *we* all are."
Their answers are:

Estelle – A kind friend
Adrienne and Barbara – A telephone friend
Geoffrey – A busy friend
Manny – An old friend
Harvey – Loyal
Ruth – Trying
Benjy – Noble

I continue, "What would our friends complain about us as friends?"

Volunteer – Being competitive
Barbara – Not listening
Daisy – Bragging

The purpose of this interaction is to create sensitivity and even empathy to the others in our relationships and to take responsibility for our behavior. We discuss this.

Warm Associations With the Word, Winter

Finally, we have a cold wintery day. Since the session on summer was so successful, I decide to do a session on winter. This is a bit more difficult. No songs come up right away and their associations are not as vivid. It takes a lot of work, on my part, to connect them to winter scenes but somehow there are interesting, vivid and moving responses.

For the warm-up, I say, "Let's hear your associations with the word winter."

Lila – winter means Florida
Brian – the winter of our discontent
Mitch – snowball fights
Lionel – ice
Me – burst pipes
Lila – taking an hour to dress the kids
Lionel – fog, chestnuts, the flu, skiing
Monica – a fireplace
Michal – slush
– coats
Barbara – sleds

I continue: "Think of a picture of yourself in the winter in our imaginary photo album." I help them connect with a brief guided imagery.

Mitch – being unable to see through my hood and jacket
Lionel – playing with my dog
Mitch – to get to school in the morning I had to take three trains through the snow.
Adrienne – 1941, during the war. We had to dig ourselves out of our house, through the snow.
Ruth – ice skating
Lila – harsh winds
Brian: The photo that comes up is on a very cold morning when I come into the kitchen . . . my mother warming me up and my father berating me.

Brian's offering is an invitation for a short vignette – a quick scene between Brian and his mother cuddling him to keep him warm. Michal, our volunteer, plays his mother based on Brian's information. Very quickly Brian recalls his papa berating him and calling him a sissy. We open this up to another short exchange between Brian and his father. Brian then takes this unexpected opportunity to say the following to his parents, "Papa, thanks for making a man out of me. Mama, thank you for loving me."

Brian has tears in his eyes. He needs this opportunity to *close* with his parents. It is definitely enough for him for now. This short interaction opens to their sharing what in their experience was the inability of fathers to express emotion.

Even Simon, who never volunteers to talk, speaks up, "My father wasn't very emotional." Most of the group nods in agreement. Everyone announces the way they referred to their parents: dad, mom, papa, mama, mommy, daddy, père, maman. They are recapturing their youth. I use this opportunity to ask them what their children called them and what their spouses called them.

The session is almost over so I ask for some winter songs and we get – Jingle Bells, Winter Wonderland and a Chanuka song. I close by saying, "When you leave today, hold onto your warm winter memories." I thank Brian for bringing us the scene of being cuddled by our mothers in the harsh cold winters. He is still smiling and it is very palpable that he still can feel his mother's warmth and care and his mother's softness.

The Essence of Life

This is a first! Why not share an interesting TED talk with our group. They are ready for this kind of intellectual stimulation. All of them! This TED talk is about a research project that started 75 years ago and is still going on. The lives of 724 men were tracked from the age of 18 and continued for 75 years to see what made them happy and healthy in their youth and how these goals changed as they faced life. The population consisted of young men from Harvard and young men from the poorer sections of Boston. When these men were young, they thought that money and fame would bring them happiness and good health.

I decide to open up this subject with our group. I tell the group about the research but I do not divulge the results of the research until they go down memory lane and share with us what was important to them at the age of 18. Only one participant in the group cannot do this. She remembers NOTHING! But she does enjoy listening to everyone else. I complicate matters by using the pillow and asking them to decide who will speak next by throwing the pillow to someone who they describe. This works beautifully because we have been doing this exercise often and they remember the instructions. It encourages and facilitates connecting. Their answers are authentic and meaningful to them. They are also very interested in hearing what others have to say. The fact that they decide who they want to hear next facilitates a direct connection and is also empowering. They are alert, involved and most important of all, they are remembering! Here are a few of their answers.

> **I ask:** When I was 18, what did I think would make me happy and healthy?
>
> **Mitch** – Not going back and forth on the subway to get to college. It was an hour and a half each way! Learning and progressing with knowledge.
>
> **Lila** – To work and make money.
>
> **Geoffrey** – To overcome my intense shyness with girls.
>
> **Brian** – A beautiful woman, a promise from a female.
>
> **Jennie** – (staff) A guy called Don.
>
> **Ruth** – I was in Israel studying. My goal was to implement everything I learned from my youth movement.
>
> **Gila** – (staff) A husband and children . . . family.
>
> **Monica** – Looking forward to a good marriage in good health for my family and it came to be. A happy home with lots of kids.
>
> **Robert** – To move to Israel.
>
> **Michal (volunteer)** – Freedom. Leaving my parents' home and seeing what life had to offer.
>
> **Herbie** – A girl.
>
> **Debra** – Nothing! (She could not think of anything despite our attempts to help her.)
>
> **Me** – The ability to create to act, perform and direct and to marry and have six children.
>
> **Ilana** – To get married and have a family (she is a newlywed social worker on internship.) Working in something that I like.
>
> **Lionel** – I was a lonely boy. I had very few friends. What I needed and didn't get was guidance. I wasn't mature enough to know what to do with my life. I was pessimistic.

I did a double for Lionel which he totally accepted: *My parents were not interested in what I wanted. They just wanted me to be a good religious boy and fulfill my duties. They guided me in what was important to THEM.*

(Thank you, TED talks for giving Lionel the opportunity to express this deep resentment.)

> **Monica** – fixing. Working in a museum, like my father, I worked in restoration.
>
> **Martin** – basketball
>
> **Adina** – (volunteer aged 18) Enjoying life. Going on trips with my friends. Cutting class.

At this point, I revealed that the research showed that after 75 years, the most important thing in life is not being alone. Having people around you. Having relationships. That's what is happening to all of us in Melabev. Everyone agreed.

> The research showed that after 75 years, the most important thing in life is not being alone. Having people around you. Having relationships.

Reaching Out for Help

In this session, I emphasize that we are *not* going to talk about the past. We are going to talk about today, the present, now. First, we explore: who do I turn to when I have a problem and then what sort of problems propel me to seek help?

Their responses are, when I have a problem and I need help, I turn to a spouse, a sibling, child, grandchild social worker, aide, technician, doctor, neighbor, friend, myself, God! I continue by asking: Who is the first person you go to when you have a problem?

Adrienne – My grandson for dealing with finances or my son-in-law in Australia.
I ask: what happens if you need someone nearby?
Daisy – My social worker.
Martin – If I need money, I go to the bank. If I need a doctor, I go to a doctor! If I have a problem, I solve it.
Lionel – For keeping up with technology I used to turn to my neighbor downstairs but now he has moved away so I turn to my brother, who lives nearby, or my grandchildren.
Herbie – If I have a problem I turn to a psychiatrist. (His situation has deteriorated immensely. He now has Lewy body dementia and suffers from hallucinations. He participates by listening with intensity and keeping himself under control.
Robert – I turn to my wife and to my kids.
Simon – I turn to my wife.
Monica, Ruth, Debra, Barbara – my children.
Geoffrey – I can't immediately reply.

Geoffrey's response is a typical example of a member of our group who wants to participate and is having trouble. This subject is important to him. I can feel that he wants to say something but his mind is blocked. Well, maybe psychodrama can help him? I offer to help him. He is amenable. I remind him of all the options that were presented, and I ask, "What about your wife? Can we talk to her?" I am standing very close to him and I can feel his self-confidence rising. He nods his head affirmatively. We do a vignette with his wife, where he asks her for help because he doesn't remember. He knows how to express this need to his wife quite well. After taking center stage in this short role reversal with our volunteer, Michal, playing his wife, he contributes a lot to the session with humor, honesty and wit. Geoffrey has so much to contribute. He wants to feel vital. He is not giving up. He feels safe, in our circle of trust, to admit that he needs help. Just saying it, is such a relief and he is able to express his frustration. Yes, it is difficult when we want to say something and it disappears. Our group can all identify with this feeling.

On the other hand, Herbie starts hallucinating for a few minutes and Martin is sleeping. There is no magic here but it is imperative to try not to give up. Moreover, it is okay to be helped on every level, even here in our psychodrama sessions.

I end the session by summarizing when, why and from whom we ask for help. There are problems with health, hygiene, finances, technology, hosting company, food and shopping. They are all valid. The subtlety of Geoffrey's vignette shows the group that we can definitely put remembering on our list.

A Psychodramatic Meeting With an Aide

I bring in three very life-like dolls. My plan is to strengthen awareness of the participants' emotional intelligence by asking them to use their wisdom that comes from their life experiences and give this newborn baby essential suggestions on how to live a healthy, dynamic and meaningful life. But . . . one of the group leaders quietly tells me that one of our new members, Estelle, is very upset and agitated because her children have decided that she needs an aide to live with her. She announces, "I have a new person in my life who is not letting me be free."

Estelle has Parkinson's. Her hands shake all the time and it is very difficult for her to express herself. If she could voice this strong statement, it must be addressed. I decide to address the subject of "aides" with the entire group and to "trust the process". The dolls can wait.

In order for Estelle not to feel alone with this issue, I open the subject by saying, "Last week, we examined who we turn to when we have a problem? This week, we will deal with what do we do when we need help? There is a difference between having a problem and needing help NOW!"

Mitch – Scream! Yell like hell!
Libby – Go to someone you love.

I ask, "What do you do if that person is not close by or not strong enough?"

Geoffrey – Come to Melabev!

I continue, "Who can help us when we need help beyond those who usually help us?" (I knew where we were heading.)

    Lila – That's when people get caregivers, an aide.

I am now where I can help Estelle.

I ask, "Who here has an aide?" Five people raise their hands. Some of the participants who have aides do not acknowledge this until later in the session when they are more involved in the activity. Estelle does not raise her hand. I continue, thinking about how to reach *her*.

I ask, "How do we feel about having an aide?"

Mitch – It could be a little demeaning. (He does not acknowledge that he has an aide but is happy to talk about it.)

Adrienne – In the evening, I need her.

Double: *I don't want to lose my independence, but sometimes I can't manage without her.*

I then ask, "What does your aide do?"

Adrienne – Everything . . . in her own time.

Double: *She organizes me and sometimes takes control.*

Adrienne – She has been with me ever since I had my accident two years ago.

I ask Michal, our volunteer, to role-play the aide.

I say, "Let's pretend that this is your aide sitting in this chair that I just put out here. What would you like to say to her?"

Brian – I don't need you.

Monica – Welcome. Thank you.

Adrienne – I'm happy I can speak Yiddish to others so you won't understand what I am saying. Also, you are always on the phone.

I say, "What should our aide here answer you? Give her the text. Give her the words that she should use to answer you." They couldn't do this. I tried. Sometimes these participants surprise us. It doesn't hurt to try, so Michal, our volunteer made up her own text.

Michal role-playing the aide – "I need to have connections to my world. I have a family. I care about you but I also care about myself and my family."

I stand behind Michal and add this double, for the aide for Estelle to hear.

I want to help you but you won't let me.

Estelle – I find my aide very invasive and intrusive.

Michal as the aide, "When I am new, it takes time for both of us to adjust."

My double: I'm here for you. Give me some time.

Lila – Don't worry, the appreciation will come.

Me – Don't worry, she'll be kind to you as she gets to know you and doesn't feel threatened.

Estelle – I feel like I am going to scream when it's the two of us alone. I was at a party late last night, and this morning, the aide woke me at 7:30 and asked why I wasn't up yet.

I want to help Estelle. Her frustration and agitation are surfacing. I ask her if I can do a double for her and she agrees.

Double: *You are all over the place. You are threatening me. I know when to get up! Don't take my independence away. Leave me alone.*

Estelle sighs. This is what she needs. The expression of her frustration in full sentences has been a major accomplishment for her. Participating in this session is a confirmation for her.

Adrienne – The aide could say I am sorry. I had good intentions.

Lila – I love my aide.

Michal role-playing role of the the aide – Thank you.

Brian – No! I don't want your help! Go about your business and I'll do mine. She's been bossing me around for forty-seven years.

I explain, "Brian, we are not talking about our spouses. We can do that in another session. This woman sitting in this chair is a caretaker, an aide."

Geoffrey – You must need to be on the phone because you must be feeling lonely.

We then proceed to do a psychodramatic scene as a rehearsal for Barbara to tell her aide not to reorganize her drawers because then she can't find the clothing she wants to wear. After this scene, Barbara has an action insight and admits to the group, "I need to have someone to yell at!" (Actually, as a result of this enactment, Barbara proceeded to look for a more congenial aide. She finds a lovely woman who becomes her best friend. We have all met her and could see her devotion when we did Zooms during the COVID-19 lockdown.)

We then discuss how to improve communication with our aides. We do a few more rehearsal enactments. Estelle is not alone. She is feeling calmer.

Celebrating the Purim Holiday

Working with the word "happiness"

Today our session is in honor of *Rosh Hodesh Adar,* the first day of the Hebrew month that ushers in happiness.

I have brought back the scarves. This time it is a much smaller number of scarves so as not to overwhelm them. The group has a good reaction to them. I place them on the floor in the center. We are a very small group because of nasty weather, and as a result, the quiet members of the group find their voice more easily. For example, Ethel has integrated beautifully and now feels comfortable with the group and with the psychodrama. Daisy actually has actually become pretty. She sits up tall. Her hump seems so much smaller and less prominent.

There are about twenty scarves. They are all bright pleasant colors. Each person picks a color that represents happiness for them. We then place them all on the floor in the center of our circle so that we, as a group, can see what happiness is for all of us. A group feeling is created with the use of a gigantic green transparent scarf. Everyone holds onto a piece of it to create a window into the sculpture of happiness on the floor.

I then start a sentence that they are asked to finish: "I am happy when . . ." When someone says something that the participants agree with, they shake the scarf so that we can see and feel everyone's attitude towards what was said.

I am happy when:

* Things work out.
* When I feel like I've helped someone.
* I'm always happy with my family.
* When the sun is shining.

I say, "Let's hear things that are more personal."

* Doing something that I like to do that has a purpose.
* Estelle – When I am doing some exercise.
* Barbara – When I get a phone call from a friend.
* Daisy – When you walk into a room where a baby is sleeping. There is nothing more peaceful.
* Monica – When my family is doing what they are supposed to do.

Experimenting With Being Someone Else

Today is a happy Jewish holiday called Purim. We celebrate this holiday with many festivities and the custom is to come in a costume. The center is open and we have our psychodrama session with a smaller group. A benefactor of the center donated fantastic props, hats and costumes for the people to use to dress up with. Our circle is colorful and engaging.

I open up the session with the following statement, "Having the opportunity to be someone else can be exciting." I give some examples and then continue, "If I could be someone else, who would I want to be?"

Mitch – Albert Einstein.
Adrienne – I'd like to be Christopher Columbus, exploring the world.
Lionel – A psychiatrist.
Geoffrey – (Wearing a beautiful king's crown and cape) The King of Hearts.
Daisy – Cher

Quite a few stated that they are happy with who they are.

I then challenge them to be somebody else for a few minutes. Everyone is given a card with a different character written on it. They have to do or say something so that we can guess who they are. The characters are from the world of fantasy and from the real world. These are the characters I chose for this group: musician, famous artist, famous movie director, famous actress, ballerina beauty queen, sick princess, ruthless king, poor beggar, handsome prince, thief, policeman, judge, successful business man, fairy god-mother, taxi driver, typical teenager, doctor.

The session does not go the way I had planned. Two of the participants do a great job of showing us, through their actions and words, who they are. Some of them just cannot do it but they are enjoying the chance to guess what is being depicted by the others in the group. So, I ask the staff to join me in portraying some of these characters. The non-performers are happy to guess. It does not bother them that they cannot perform the task. This is important information for me. They are simply happy to participate in a stimulating activity

I hope that the detailed documentation earlier of moving sessions has given you, the reader, triggers, insights, options for activities and subjects to pursue with the people under your care or with your relatives and friends who need stimulation in order to function better in their daily routines. The people I have been working with spend a few hours a day at the daycare center. But what happens to their cognition when they are at home? Even though their family members might be available to supply their physical needs, our population of people suffering from various forms of dementia basically have a lonely existence at home. They are afraid to make mistakes. It is easier to simply withdraw and close their eyes, ears and minds. These are wake-up exercises that will induce involvement and self-efficacy.

> The people I have been working with spend a few hours a day at the daycare center. But what happens to their cognition when they are at home?

This elaboration of sessions contains gems of authentic expressions filled with wisdom, charm, insight and dignity. They will help to understand the dilemmas, conflicts, frustrations, joys, achievements and the potential of this population.

An important rationale behind the subjects I chose to bring to our sessions is what are the themes that will stimulate personal expression and social cohesion. After five years, we covered almost everything related to their lives. There were times that the subject matter was based on the here and now. At other times, they were connected to the calendar, current events near and far, or emotions that needed therapy.

Summary of Practical Applications

- Reading the documentation of various sessions is not only delightful reading, it also gives essential information on the ability of the participants to respond authentically.
  We learn something new and important about our group members in every session.
- When faced with an immediate need, the leader's spontaneity must rise to the occasion. Plans for a specific session can wait and the subject can change accordingly.
- The progression of a session also requires flexibility and spontaneity.

More Topics That Evoked Responses and Interaction

Following are subjects that were planned and subjects that arose spontaneously and subjects that this population was able to relate to easily.

What choices do we have?
I choose to . . .
What choices have I made.
What makes you satisfied with yourself?

What advice would you give to children under 10, teenagers, newly-weds, people with illnesses, new immigrants, people who are diagnosed with Alzheimer's disease, new members at Melabev?
What is friendship for you?
Let's explore the word "stubbornness".
When should we say to ourselves "so what?"
What do you want your grandchild to know about the life you have lived?
What do you wish for in the New Year?
What do we want to say goodbye to in the past year?
What do you want to give and what do you want to take from someone in the group?
What are my strengths?
A decision that you made that was significant.
Decisions you have to make now.
I would like to reconnect with . . .
When were you courageous?
It is easy for me to. . . . It is difficult for me . . .
I am lucky that . . . I am unlucky that
Heroes in my life.
Miracles in my life.
What do you need from this group?
Let's talk about longing or missing someone.
Let a person in your life or an object or a part of your body tell us something about you, perhaps even complain about you or give you a compliment.
What would you like to say to . . . a president, a politician, any sort of leader or famous person?
Rehearsing through role reversal for an important conversation with someone in our life, such as a doctor, social worker, aide, neighbor, family member or friend.
The school year is starting. Let's show our appreciation to a teacher from your childhood; someone who has influenced you significantly.
What adjectives would people in your life (like this same teacher) give you?
Be a *double* for someone new in our group. What is this new member feeling but not saying?
How often do we say the word "no"?
I am relieved when . . .
I get depressed when . . .
I feel liberated when . . . I feel enslaved when . . .
I have to accept that . . .
What do I do to feel calm?

What do we take for granted?

When are we taken for granted?

I am/was defiant when . . .

I want . . . I need . . . I should . . . I have . . . I can't . . . I can . . .
I don't . . . I wish . . . I shouldn't . . . I must . . . Don't . . . Please . . .
I hope . . .

Imaginary photo albums for every subject. Example: We are making a "PROUD" photo album. Show me what you look like when you are proud; I will photograph you. Can you tell us of a situation where you felt proud? What words should we put under this photograph to describe the situation?

Photograph albums from every stage in our lives.

Something that I have to forgive myself for.

What do I have in common with my parents?

What do I have in common with my children?

We invited Dr. Alzheimer to our session so that he or she could give the group essential information about the disease.

Good deeds day – tell us about a good deed that you did and one that someone did for you.

An accomplishment you are proud of.

What trait am I proud of?

What trait helps me cope with my situation?

What trait would I like to change, improve or get rid of?

An embarrassing or funny situation that happened to me.

Let's talk about marriage. This leads to talking about divorce.

What do I take from this session?

What do I want to throw away or leave from this session?

Example: I take encouragement and I leave despair.

I am sure you can add many more subjects. In a group filled with trust, holding, safety and sharing, most subjects are appropriate.

More About Melabev, a Jerusalem Daycare Center for Dementia and the Elderly

Dr. Zeev Friedman, the CEO of Melabev, writes:

Melabev, a unique non-profit organization in Israel established forty years ago, specializes in dementia and the care of Alzheimer in the community. It was established in 1981 by a gerontologist, Professor Arnold Rosin, OBM, head of the Geriatric Department of the Shaare Zedek Medical Center, Jerusalem, and another geriatric social worker Leah Abramowitz. Together they opened Melabev's first day center and worked tirelessly to design unique programs and therapeutic activities that engage the participants, exercising their mind, body, and soul, and thus infusing purpose to their lives.

Melabev operates four multi-lingual day centers for Hebrew, Russian, French, English, and Arabic speakers. Communicating with a person in their mother tongue is essential for them socially, helping them feel their needs are met, and they are understood and safe. The day centers in Jerusalem and Beit Shemesh serve persons experiencing the effects of dementia or Alzheimer's in every cognitive level – mildly impaired, moderately impaired, and severely impaired (low functioning).

Beyond caring for someone in cognitive and memory decline, Melabev supports primary caregivers and family members. Support groups are an integral part of serving the whole family.

In addition, Melabev offers therapy services in the home and professional caregiver services in other parts of Israel. For further information, call Melabev at 1-700-70-4533 or refer to the Melabev website at www.melabev.org.

Glossary of Terms and Elaborations

The following are explanations of the technical terms used throughout the book as applied to my work and as necessarily simplified for work with this population. The main sources for the official definitions or explanations that are quoted here are derived from these authors: Anne Ancelin-Schutzenberger, Rene F. Marineau, Adam Blatner and J.L. Moreno.

Action Insight

Action insight is the result of various kinds of action learning. It may be defined as the integration of emotional, cognitive, imaginary, behavioral and interpersonal learning experiences . . . (It) cannot be attained through introspective analysis while lying on the couch. It is achieved only in action while moving about, standing still, pushing and pulling, making sounds or gestures . . . (it) may appear as a sudden flash of comprehension – Eureka! I've got it! – or as the gradual unfolding of discoveries.

(Kellerman, 1992, p. 86)

Auxiliary Ego A person in the circle of participants who is *chosen* to portray someone or something in the psychodramatic scene we are enacting. The text for the auxiliary is supplied by the participant and is his or her directed, *heard* voice. In our group, we were fortunate enough to have a volunteer to play the part of the auxiliary ego whenever necessary.

Concretizing Using a concrete object to give shape and form to a person's intrapsychic expression. In our group, I used the scarves, photos and objects from my basket or from the center.

Double This is the unheard voice of the protagonist. I say, "I am going to try and say out loud what I think you are feeling but not saying." I ask for permission to do this. Our group loves getting and listening to doubles. It strengthens their innate feelings and finds the words, phrases and sentences that they can no longer retrieve or organize on account of their dementia. I usually ask them to repeat the part of the double that they identify with.

Empty Chair   A technique in psychodrama where the director places an empty chair in the center of the circle in order to develop an enactment or simply help the clients express some deeply rooted issues or unfinished business. In our group I would say, "Imagine so and so or some item or part of your body is sitting in this chair. What would you like to say to him or her or it?"

Enactment   In psychodrama, we do, we show and want to see what's happening. We experience! Rather than just telling, we need to *show* what we're feeling. We can do this through acting out a scene in our life or even rehearsing for a scene that we need to experience. We can set up a scene and be there and remember. We can do role-playing and role reversals. Using the technique of photo albums, we can reenact scenes from our lives the way Martin did in the section called LOVE. The scenes can be past, present or future. They can be real or imaginary. Moreno summarizes this so well, and suggests that psychodrama be applied in the very situation and place where the conflict occurs, whether in the home, schoolyard, at work or on the street . . . He felt that Freud saw his patients in an artificial setting. In psychodrama, even though the action takes place on the stage, a good deal of time is taken for the protagonist to recapture the concrete elements of the setting, and he or she is invited to describe them in exact detail for an authentic experiential replay of the scene.

Mirroring   In psychodrama, the protagonist may be unable to represent himself, or the director may want the protagonist to see himself from another perspective. He goes out of the scene and stands or sits in a place where he has a full view of an auxiliary ego portraying him. By re-enacting and copying his behavior and trying to express his feelings in words and movement, the auxiliary gives the protagonist an objective mirrored view of himself. It allows the protagonist to witness the scene from the side.

Protagonist   The person in the group who is exploring or working on an issue and is the focus of the enactment.

Role Reversal   The protagonist plays the role of the other in the scene and an auxiliary ego portrays him. The roles are constantly reversed. In this technique, the person can better understand what the other person is feeling and experiencing. In our group, we were fortunate to have a volunteer, who was interested in psychodrama, take on the roles when necessary. (De-roling is when the person playing the other, announces at the end of the enactment, that she is not the person depicted, she is ____ and announces her name.)

Sharing   This is a psychodramatic technique where we talk about ourselves and about how we have connected to what we have just witnessed in the enactment. When the other participants talk about their experiences, the protagonist feels less exposed and alone. The group members are united through profound emotional expression and identifying.

Sociodrama   is the use of psychodrama tools to give expression to an issue that the participants share, such as elections or current events.

Sociometry   a measurement of interpersonal relationships. In our group I used this term instead of the term "spectrogram". It was easier for them to interpret this word.

Spectogram   A technique in psychodrama where the group can see the dynamics of the various feelings in a group. The director defines the two poles on the spectrum of an issue and has the group show by positioning themselves on an axis from 0 to 10 where they "stand" on this particular issue. In our group, we did this by raising our hands from 0 on their lap to 10 high up in the air, since there was no way the members of this group could stand.

Surplus Reality   This technique enables us to go beyond and transcend reality. We can talk to and be anyone or anything anywhere. We can take advantage of this technique in order to communicate with someone close to us who has passed away. It makes it possible to re-enact a scene and change the ending. Most of our participants were sophisticated enough to appreciate the understanding that we have alternatives in how we perceive a situation. We can alter the way we or someone else has actually behaved!

We can be in the future or in the past. We can imagine ourselves in any situation. The opportunities are endless. These sessions can be fun, idyllic, powerful, meaningful and emotional. *Surplus reality* is the "term given to the enactment of events which never happened and never can happen, the voicing of words never said" (Wilkins p. 32). I have found the use of surplus reality very helpful in issues of unfinished business. It also enables our participants to understand the views, attitudes and behavior of people in their lives past and present and sometimes, even future. Some aspects of surplus reality are called *future projection* where we can imagine and enact a change that we would like to see in the future.

Tele   This is Greek meaning "far" or "far off" and Moreno calls it "distance" and describes it as "the simplest unit of feeling transmitted from one individual to another" (Moreno, 1953, p. 159). It is the process of interaction between individuals. Kellerman says that, unlike empathy, it is a two-way flow of feeling. Tian Dayton explains this subtle but powerful situation explicitly. She writes: "We have all met people whom we seem to know and understand immediately, without even speaking. We encounter people with whom we are instinctively comfortable. . . . It is a sort of telepathic sensory awareness" (Dayton, 1994, 28–29).

Tele in our group occurred many times. The staff certainly was communicating non-verbally in many instances. Tele occurs when I know that a statement made by one of our participants has to be opened up and developed into a psychodrama. I look at that person and our eyes meet. I know it is okay to ask that person if we can psychodramatically meet the person he or she is talking about. They know this will lead to an action insight and help the relationship heal. It even occurs between members on many circumstances. When Deena spoke about her love for her son who had just passed away from cancer, Brian got up and walked over to her and kissed her on the forehead. He said, "I love you." That was enough. The connection was much deeper than an ordinary touch or word. He had to approach her. He had to touch her. He knew what she was feeling and he also knew that she needed his kiss through *tele* between them. The way she accepted this was her reciprocation to him. It was a "moment".

When the group waits patiently for someone to organize their words and make their statement, it comes from respect but it also is a form of tele. It is a non-verbal understanding. The group knows that the speaker needs the time to put his or her thoughts together and the speaker knows that the group wants to hear his or her sentence and is not pressured to hurry. It is mutual and helps us understand this delicate sensitivity and non-verbal communication.

As a student studying psychodrama, I experienced tele. Zerka Moreno (Moreno's widow) was invited to spend a day with us. She demonstrated an entire psychodrama session with all of the students in our program. It was a three-hour workshop. At one point in the psychodrama enactment, I was very excited because I felt that I would have done exactly what Zerka had done with the protagonist. I was uplifted and exhilarated by the notion. After the workshop, she came over to me and said, "I felt a tele with you in this session." She was correct!

Back to our population. When you think about it, tele is a subtle but powerful connection. For this population to be able to reach this level of trust, unconscious connection and understanding is an achievement I did not even dare to put in my list of goals. It was subtle but it did exist.

Vignette   A scene. This specific population cannot go through the entire psychodrama curve. We can open up an issue to a short enactment.

Bibliography

Alexander, F., and French, T. (1946) *Psychoanalytic Theory: Principles and Application*. New York: Ronald Press.

Bailey, S.D. (1993) *Wings to Fly*. Rockville, MD: Woodbine House.

Blatner, A. (1996). *Acting-in: Practical Applications of Psychodramatic Methods*. 3rd edition. New York: Springer.

Blatner, A., with Blatner, A. (1988) *Foundations of Psychodrama: History, Theory and Practice*. 3rd edition. New York: Springer.

Blatner, A.M.D., and Blatner, A. (2007) *The Art of Play: Helping Adults Reclaim Imagination and Spontaneity*. Revised edition. New York: Brunner/Mazel and Human Sciences.

Bolton, G. (1984) *Drama as Education*. Essex: Longman.

Brown, N., Cedar, T., and Tziraki, C. (2022). Psychodrama with Persons with Dementia on Zoom: Proof of Concept. *Dementia: The International Journal of Social Research and Practice*, 21(4): 1289–1303.

Caldwell, L., and Joyce, A. (eds.) (2012) *Reading Winnicott*. New York: Routledge.

Chesner, A. (1995) *Dramatherapy for People with Learning Disabilities*. London: Jessica Kingsley Publishers.

Cottrell, J. (1987) *Teaching with Creative Dramatics*. Lincolnwood, IL: National Textbook Co.

Dayton, T. (1994) *The Drama within*. Deerfield Beach, FL: Health Communications, Inc.

Dayton, T. (2005) *The Living Stage: A Step-by-Step Guide to Psychodrama and Experiential Group Therapy*. Deerfield Beach, FL: Health Communications, Inc.

Emunah, R. (1994) *Acting for Real; Drama Therapy Process, Technique, and Performance*. New York: Brunner/Mazel.

Fox, J. (ed.) (1987) *The Essential Moreno: Writings on Psychodrama, Group Method and Spontaneity by J.L. Moreno, MD*. New York: Springer.

Gershoni, J. (ed.) (2003) *Psychodrama in the 21st Century: Clinical and Educational Application*. New York: Springer.

Gersie, A. (1996) *Dramatic Approaches to Brief Therapy*. London, Bristol and Pennsylvania: Jessica Kingsley.

Goren-Bar, A. (1993) Three Self Theories, in H. Kohut, D. Stern, and C. Bollas (eds.) *Applied to Intermodal Expressive Therapy* (Doctoral Dissertation). Cincinnati, OH: Union Institute [pub. in University Microfilm Inc., May, 1955]

Hartnoll, P. (1985) *The Theater; A Concise History*. Revised edition. New York: Thames and Hudson.

Hoey, B. (1997) *Who Calls the Tune? A Psychodramatic Approach to Child Therapy*. London and New York: Routledge.

Hollander, C. (1969) *A Process for Psychodrama Training: The Hollander Psychodrama Curve*. Littleton, CO: Evergreen Institute Press.

Holmes, P. (1992) *The Inner World Outside: Object Relations Theory and Psychodrama*. London and New York: Routledge.

Holmes, P., Karp, M., and Watson, M. (eds.). (1994) *Psychodrama since Moreno: Innovations in Theory and Practice*. London: Routledge.

Jennings, S. (1973) *Remedial Drama*. Great Britain: Pitman Press.

Jennings, S. (ed.) (1987) *Dramatherapy; Theory and Practice for Teachers and Clinicians*. Cambridge, MA: Brookline Books.

Johnson, D., Pendzik, S., and Snow, S. (eds.) (2012) *Assessment in Drama Therapy*. Springfield, IL: Charles C. Thomas.

Kahn, M. (1997) *Between Therapist and Client: A New Relationship*. New York: Freeman.

Kaisaris, S., Gesser-Edelsburg, A., Yaniv, D., and Palgi, Y. (2020). Playback Theatre in Adult Day Centers: A Creative Group Intervention for Community-dwelling Older Adults. *PLoS ONE*, 15(10): e0239812. https://doi.org/10.1371/journal.pone.0239812.

Karp, M. (1994) The River of Freedom, in P. Holmes, M. Karp, and M. Watson (eds.) *Psychodrama since Moreno: Innovations in Theory and Practice*. London and New York: Routledge.

Karp, M. (1998) An Introduction to Psychodrama, in M. Karp, P. Holmes, and K.B. Tauvon (eds.) *The Handbook of Psychodrama*. London: Routledge.

Karp, M., Holmes, P., and Bradshaw Tauvon, K. (eds.) (1998) *The Handbook of Psychodrama*. London and New York: Routledge.

Kedem-Tahar, E., and Kellerman, P.F. (1996) Psychodrama and Dramatherapy: A Comparison. *The Arts in Psychotherapy*, 23(1): 27–36.

Kellerman, P.F. (1979) Transference, Countertransference and Tele. *Journal of Group Psychotherapy, Psychodrama and Sociometry*, 32: 38–55.

Kellerman, P.F. (1992) *Focus on Psychodrama*. London: Jessica Kingsley.

Kellerman, P.F., and Hudgins, M.K. (eds.) (2000) *Psychodrama with Trauma Survivors: Acting Out Your Pain*. London: Jessica Kingsley.

Kipper, D.A. (1986). *Psychotherapy through Clinical Roleplaying*. New York: Brunner/Mazel.

Kligerman, C. (1983) Art and the Self of the Artist, in A. Goldberg (ed.) *Advances in Self-Psychology* (pp. 383–396). London: Jessica Kingsley, International Universities Press.

Kohut, H. (1971) *Analysis of the Self*. New York, NY: International Universities Press.

Kohut, H. (1977) *The Restoration of the Self*. New York, NY: International Universities Press.

Kohut, H. (1978) *The Search for Self: Selective Writings of Heinz Kohut*. Madison, CT: International Universities Press.

Kohut, H., Goldberg, A., and Stepansky, P. (eds.) (1984) *How Does Analysis Cure?* Chicago, IL: The University of Chicago Press.

Landy, R. (1993) *Persona and Performance: The Meaning of Role in Theater Therapy and Everyday Life*. New York: Guilford.

Landy, R. (1994) *Drama Therapy: Concepts and Practices*. Springfield, IL: C.C. Thomas.

Landy, R., and Butler, J.D. (2012) Assessment through Role Theory, in D. Johnson, S. Pendzik, and S. Snow (eds.) *Assessment in Drama Therapy.* Springfield, IL: Charles C. Thomas.

Langley, D.M. (1983) *Dramatherapy and Psychiatry.* London: Croom Helm.

Lerner, J. (1997) *Learning Disabilities; Theory, Diagnosis and Teaching Strategies.* 7th edition. Boston, MA: Houghton Mifflin Co.

Mace, N., and Rabins, P. (2011) *The 36 Hour Day Fifth Edition; A Family Guide to Caring for People Who Have Alzheimer Disease, Related Dementias, and Memory Loss.* Baltimore, MD: The Johns Hopkins University Press.

MacIntyre, A. (2007) *After Virtue: A Study in Moral Theology.* 3rd edition. Notre Dame, IN: University of Notre Dame Press.

Mc Leod, J.N. (1978) *Some Curriculum Implications of Teaching Drama.* Carlton: Drama Resource Centre, Victoria Education Dept.

Mc Niff, S. (1981) *The Arts and Psychotherapy.* Springfield, IL: Charles C. Thomas.

Moreno, J.L. (1953) *Who Shall Survive?* New York: Beacon House.

Moreno, J.L. (1985) *The Autobiography of J. L. Moreno, M.D.* (abridged) (J.L. Moreno, Moreno Archives). Cambridge, MA: Harvard University.

Morgan, N., and Saxton, J. (1989) *Teaching Drama.* Great Britain: Stanley Thornes.

Rowe, C.E., and Mac Isaac, D.S. (1989) *Empathic Attunement: The Technique of Psychoanalytic Self Psychology,* New Jersey: Jason Aaronson.

Sacks, J. (2019) *Covenant and Conversation, Deuteronomy: Renewal of the Sinai Covenant.* Jerusalem: Maggid Books.

Sacks, J. (2020) *Judaism's Life-Changing Ideas.* Jerusalem: Maggid Books.

Siegel, A.M. (1996) *Heinz Kohut and the Psychology of the Self.* London and New York: Routledge.

Siks, G.B. (1977) *Drama with Children.* New York: Harper and Row.

Spolin, V. (1986) *Theater Games for the Classroom: A Teacher's Handbook.* Evanston, IL: Northwestern University Press.

Stanford, G., and Roark, A. (1974) *Human Interaction in Education.* Boston, MA: Allyn and Bacon.

Twitchell, D. (1978) *Social Learning in the Schools through Psychodrama.* Maine: Old Town Teacher's Corps.

Wagner, B. (1976) *Dorothy Heathcote: Drama as a Learning Medium.* Washington, DC: National Education Association.

Way, B. (1967) *Development through Drama.* Atlantic Highlands, NJ: Humanities Press.

Wilkins, P. (1999) *Psychodrama.* Los Angeles, CA: SAGE Publications Inc.

Williams, A. (1989) *The Passionate Technique.* London and New York: Routledge.

Winnicott, D. (1986) *Home Is Where We Start From.* Great Britain: Penguin.

Wolf, E. (1996) The Viennese Chicagoan, in Siegel M. Allen (ed.) *Heinz Kohut and the Psychology of the Self.* London and New York: Routledge.

Yalom, I. (1985) *The Theory and Practice of Group Psychotherapy.* 3rd edition. New York: Basic Books.

Yaniv, D. (2018). Trust the Process: A New Scientific Outlook on Psychodramatic Spontaneity Training. *Frontiers in Psychology,* 9. www.frontiersin.org/article/ 10.3389/fpsyg.2018.02083. doi.org/10.3389/fpsyg.2018.020.

Index

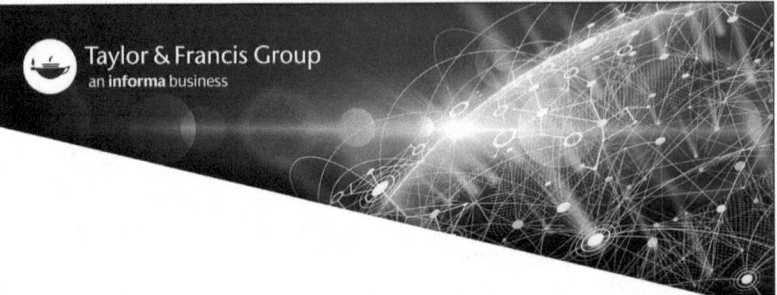
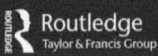
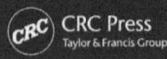